PSYCHIATRY - THEORY, APPLICATIONS AND TREATMENTS

OBSESSIVE-COMPULSIVE DISORDER

SYMPTOMS, THERAPY AND CLINICAL CHALLENGES

PSYCHIATRY - THEORY, APPLICATIONS AND TREATMENTS

Additional books and e-books in this series can be found on Nova's website under the Series tab.

PSYCHIATRY - THEORY, APPLICATIONS AND TREATMENTS

OBSESSIVE-COMPULSIVE DISORDER

SYMPTOMS, THERAPY AND CLINICAL CHALLENGES

JEFFREY L. NELSON
EDITOR

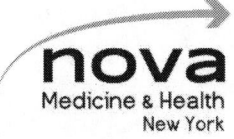

Copyright © 2021 by Nova Science Publishers, Inc.
DOI: https://doi.org/10.52305/PLHB7934

All rights reserved. No part of this book may be reproduced, stored in a retrieval system or transmitted in any form or by any means: electronic, electrostatic, magnetic, tape, mechanical photocopying, recording or otherwise without the written permission of the Publisher.

We have partnered with Copyright Clearance Center to make it easy for you to obtain permissions to reuse content from this publication. Simply navigate to this publication's page on Nova's website and locate the "Get Permission" button below the title description. This button is linked directly to the title's permission page on copyright.com. Alternatively, you can visit copyright.com and search by title, ISBN, or ISSN.

For further questions about using the service on copyright.com, please contact:
Copyright Clearance Center
Phone: +1-(978) 750-8400   Fax: +1-(978) 750-4470   E-mail: info@copyright.com.

NOTICE TO THE READER

The Publisher has taken reasonable care in the preparation of this book, but makes no expressed or implied warranty of any kind and assumes no responsibility for any errors or omissions. No liability is assumed for incidental or consequential damages in connection with or arising out of information contained in this book. The Publisher shall not be liable for any special, consequential, or exemplary damages resulting, in whole or in part, from the readers' use of, or reliance upon, this material. Any parts of this book based on government reports are so indicated and copyright is claimed for those parts to the extent applicable to compilations of such works.

Independent verification should be sought for any data, advice or recommendations contained in this book. In addition, no responsibility is assumed by the Publisher for any injury and/or damage to persons or property arising from any methods, products, instructions, ideas or otherwise contained in this publication.

This publication is designed to provide accurate and authoritative information with regard to the subject matter covered herein. It is sold with the clear understanding that the Publisher is not engaged in rendering legal or any other professional services. If legal or any other expert assistance is required, the services of a competent person should be sought. FROM A DECLARATION OF PARTICIPANTS JOINTLY ADOPTED BY A COMMITTEE OF THE AMERICAN BAR ASSOCIATION AND A COMMITTEE OF PUBLISHERS.

Additional color graphics may be available in the e-book version of this book.

Library of Congress Cataloging-in-Publication Data

ISBN: 978-1-68507-310-7

Published by Nova Science Publishers, Inc. † New York

CONTENTS

Preface		vii
Chapter 1	Obsessive-Compulsive Disorder: A General Overview *Riccardo Santini, Antonella Mariano, Federico Fiori Nastro, Martina Pelle, Alberto Siracusano, Cinzia Niolu and Flavia di Michele*	1
Chapter 2	Relevant Mechanisms in Treating Obsessive-Compulsive Disorder: The Case for Domain-Specific Relevance with Scrupulosity and Other Forms of Obsessions and Compulsions *Dakota Mauzay*	57
Chapter 3	Acute-Onset Subtypes of Pediatric Obsessive-Compulsive Disorder: Pediatric Acute-Onset Neuropsychiatric Syndrome and Pediatric Autoimmune Neuropsychiatric Disorders Associated with Streptococcal Infections *Canan Kuygun Karci*	89

Chapter 4	The Effects of COVID-19 Pandemic on Children and Adolescents with Obsessive-Compulsive Disorder *Canan Kuygun Karci*	**111**
Chapter 5	A Review of Considerations in Assessing and Treating Religious-Themed Obsessions *Kelly N. Banneyer*	**125**
Index		**137**

PREFACE

Obsessive-compulsive disorder (OCD), which is characterized by distressing intrusive thoughts and repetitive, time-consuming, task-oriented actions intended to counter these thoughts and reduce anxiety, represents a serious psychiatric condition and cause of disability worldwide. This book consists of five chapters that provide details on the effects of OCD and strategies for reducing its negative impact. Chapter one provides a general overview of OCD, including its neurochemical basis and treatment approaches. Chapter two explores some of the nuisances present in working with individuals with OCD within the context of obsessive and compulsive content that may require additive elements to be considered in treatment. Chapter three discusses the diagnostic criteria, clinical aspects, and current treatment approaches of pediatric acute-onset neuropsychiatric syndrome and pediatric autoimmune neuropsychiatric disorders associated with streptococcal infections. Chapter four describes the effects of the COVID-19 pandemic on children and adolescents with OCD. Lastly, chapter five explains the role that religion takes in certain presentations of OCD and informs clinicians how to differentiate between standard religious practices and compulsive behaviors.

Chapter 1 - Obsessive compulsive disorder (OCD) is a serious multifactorial psychiatric illness with a lifetime prevalence of 2-3%. It is characterized by distressing intrusive thoughts (obsessions), and task-oriented repetitive, time-consuming actions (compulsions) planned to contrast these thoughts and decrease the amount of anxiety. Typical compulsive behaviors include excessive hand-washing, repetitive checking, and concern for order and symmetry. OCD begins in late adolescence or early adulthood, although also children can be affected by an autoimmune OCD syndrome (PANDAS). OCD presents often in comorbidity with other psychiatric disorders, such as anxiety disorders, major depression, impulse control disorders and attention deficit disorders. A substantial risk of suicide in OCD patients is now well recognized. Therefore, the burden of disease is very high and OCD represents a leading cause of disability. The pathophysiology of OCD is extremely complex and heterogeneous, a dysfunction in the cortico-striatal-thalamo-cortical circuit seems to be the core. Recent hypotheses placing OCD in the context of impulsive control disorders in a trans-diagnostic fashion that includes basal impulse dysregulation, suggest an impaired reward and punishment processing with attenuated dopamine release in the ventral striatum. Moreover, a dysfunction in the glutamatergic neurotransmission, as well as neuroimmune abnormalities might be involved in the pathophysiology of this disorder. Due to the heterogeneity of OCD neurobiology, assessing the quantitative EEG of OCD patients could be useful before deciding about treatment strategy and for predicting treatment response. Treatment approaches range from the use of medications to cognitive behavioral therapy, non-invasive brain stimulation (TMS), to surgery. The use of antidepressants, such as tricyclics or serotonin reuptake inhibitors, is based on the involvement of the serotonergic system and the reduction of the anxiety rate in OCD. Atypical antipsychotics represent another class of medications used in the management of OCD symptoms, often in add-on with antidepressants. The alterations in signaling and metabolism of glutamate suggest the use of glutamate-modulating agents. Nutraceutics with anti-inflammatory, neuromodulatory and neuroprotective activity may represent a complementary useful treatment for OCD, considering the evidence-based problem of treatment resistance. Nutraceutics must be also considered for treatment of special populations such as young population and elders. Despite significant therapeutic advances, there remain several challenges in treating OCD. Integrated understanding of the pathophysiology of OCD in the context of dimensional psychiatry and future directions for research will be discussed in the chapter.

Chapter 2 - Contrary to popular representations of obsessive-compulsive disorder (OCD), OCD is a highly heterogeneous presentation. As such, there are a variety of clinical constructs and hypothesized mechanisms of action clinicians need to consider when working with OCD. This is of paramount importance as the body of knowledge within the treatment literature of OCD grows and continued differences between symptom subtypes of OCD are observed. Indeed, it is possible that varying presentations of OCD may have different mechanisms of action. Further, personal and cultural factors have been articulated as being relevant to the treatment of differing subtypes of OCD. Although there is a growing body of evidence indicating some treatments can be a highly effective means of treating OCD, it is important to note that even highly effective treatments often leave many still suffering from their obsessions and compulsions. Further, the possibility for homogeneous treatments of OCD to result in a "one size fits all" mentality necessitates continued attention being given to the aforementioned areas of OCD discussed. The present writing explores some of the nuisances present in working with individuals with OCD within the context of obsessive and compulsive content that may require additive elements to be considered in treatment. Particular attention is given to scrupulosity and factors relevant within the treatment of scrupulosity.

Chapter 3 - Pediatric acute-onset neuropsychiatric syndrome (PANS) and pediatric autoimmune neuropsychiatric disorders associated with streptococcal infections (PANDAS) are acute-onset subtypes of obsessive-compulsive disorder (OCD) in children. PANDAS include sudden-onset OCD symptoms and new-onset tics due to streptococcal infection. PANDAS were first defined by Swedo in 1998. In 2012, a new diagnostic criterion (PANS) was proposed for patients who met all

PANDAS criteria except for association with streptococcal infection. For the diagnosis of PANS, sudden-onset OCD symptoms and/or severe food restriction are accompanied by at least two of the following: depression/emotional lability, anxiety, irritability, aggression and/or oppositional behavior, behavioral regression, somatic symptoms, deteriorated school performance, and sensorimotor abnormalities required. Although it is hypothesized that the pathogenesis of PANDAS and Sydenham's chorea is similar, definitive proof of the pathogenesis is lacking. Also, there are many unresolved questions about diagnostic criteria and the clinical approach for PANS/PANDAS. This creates confusion and difficulty in treatment and follow-up. In this chapter, the diagnostic criteria, clinical aspects, and current treatment approaches of PANDAS and PANS will be discussed.

Chapter 4 - The past one year has been difficult for people around the world in a way that has not been experienced before. Studies examining the effects of the COVID-19 pandemic are increasing day by day. It is known that traumas and difficult life events may trigger or worsen obsessive-compulsive disorder (OCD) symptoms. Numerous studies with adult OCD patients have reported that these patients are more vulnerable to COVID-19-related stress and their OCD symptoms worsened also new obsessions and compulsions developed during the COVID-19 pandemic. There are very few studies in the literature investigating the effects of the COVID-19 pandemic on children and adolescents with OCD. In this chapter, the effects of the COVID-19 pandemic on children and adolescents with OCD will be discussed.

Chapter 5 - OCD oftentimes can target an individual's values. For those individuals of a strong faith background, scrupulosity can become a focus of intrusive thoughts. Scrupulosity may involve intrusive thoughts related to blasphemy, having committed a sin, behaving morally, purity, going to Hell, death, or a loss of control. 24.8% of adults and 37.7% of children with OCD have religious obsessions, and these obsessions can vary across religious groups. Compulsions associated with these behaviors can include confessing, seeking reassurance, cleansing and purifying rituals, excessive prayer, and avoidance of triggers. This chapter will explain the role that religion takes in certain presentations of OCD and inform clinicians how to differentiate between standard religious practices and compulsive behaviors. In working within an exposure-based cognitive behavioral model for intervention, this chapter will also discuss implications for evidence-based treatment using a case example.

In: Obsessive-Compulsive Disorder
Editor: Jeffrey L. Nelson

ISBN: 978-1-68507-310-7
© 2021 Nova Science Publishers, Inc.

Chapter 1

OBSESSIVE-COMPULSIVE DISORDER: A GENERAL OVERVIEW

Riccardo Santini[1], MD, Antonella Mariano[1], MD, Federico Fiori Nastro[1], MD, Martina Pelle[1], MD, Alberto Siracusano[1,2], MD, Cinzia Niolu[1,2], MD and Flavia di Michele[2,*], MD, PhD

[1]Tor Vergata University, Rome, Italy
[2]Acute Psychiatric Unit, PTV Foundation - Policlinico Tor Vergata, Rome, Italy

ABSTRACT

Obsessive compulsive disorder (OCD) is a serious multifactorial psychiatric illness with a lifetime prevalence of 2-3%. It is characterized by distressing intrusive thoughts (obsessions), and task-oriented repetitive, time-consuming actions (compulsions) planned to contrast these thoughts and decrease the amount of anxiety. Typical

---

[*] Corresponding Author's E-mail: flaviadimichele@gmail.com.

compulsive behaviors include excessive hand-washing, repetitive checking, and concern for order and symmetry. OCD begins in late adolescence or early adulthood, although also children can be affected by an autoimmune OCD syndrome (PANDAS). OCD presents often in comorbidity with other psychiatric disorders, such as anxiety disorders, major depression, impulse control disorders and attention deficit disorders. A substantial risk of suicide in OCD patients is now well recognized. Therefore, the burden of disease is very high and OCD represents a leading cause of disability.

The pathophysiology of OCD is extremely complex and heterogeneous, a dysfunction in the cortico-striatal-thalamo-cortical circuit seems to be the core. Recent hypotheses placing OCD in the context of impulsive control disorders in a trans-diagnostic fashion that includes basal impulse dysregulation, suggest an impaired reward and punishment processing with attenuated dopamine release in the ventral striatum. Moreover, a dysfunction in the glutamatergic neurotransmission, as well as neuroimmune abnormalities might be involved in the pathophysiology of this disorder.

Due to the heterogeneity of OCD neurobiology, assessing the quantitative EEG of OCD patients could be useful before deciding about treatment strategy and for predicting treatment response.

Treatment approaches range from the use of medications to cognitive behavioral therapy, non-invasive brain stimulation (TMS), to surgery. The use of antidepressants, such as tricyclics or serotonin reuptake inhibitors, is based on the involvement of the serotonergic system and the reduction of the anxiety rate in OCD. Atypical antipsychotics represent another class of medications used in the management of OCD symptoms, often in add-on with antidepressants. The alterations in signaling and metabolism of glutamate suggest the use of glutamate-modulating agents. Nutraceutics with anti-inflammatory, neuromodulatory and neuroprotective activity may represent a complementary useful treatment for OCD, considering the evidence-based problem of treatment resistance. Nutraceutics must be also considered for treatment of special populations such as young population and elders. Despite significant therapeutic advances, there remain several challenges in treating OCD. Integrated understanding of the pathophysiology of OCD in the context of dimensional psychiatry and future directions for research will be discussed in the chapter.

ABBREVIATIONS

5-HT	specific serotoninergic receptors (5-HT)
ACC	anterior cingulate cortex (ACC).
BD	bipolar disorder (BD)
CBT	cognitive-behavioral therapy (CBT)
CSF	cerebrospinal fluid (CSF)
CSTC	cortico-striato-thalamo-cortical (CSTC)
DBS	deep brain stimulation (DBS)
DMN	default mode network (DMN)
dTMS	deep TMS (dTMS)
ERP	exposure/response prevention (ERP)
GPe	globus pallidus (GPe)
GPi	internal globus pallidus (GPi)
ICD	impulse control disorders (ICD)
MDD	Major Depression Disorder (MDD)
NAC	N-acetyl cysteine (NAC)
NAc	nucleus accumbens (NAc)
OCD	Obsessive compulsive disorder (OCD)
OCRDs	obsessive-compulsive and related disorders (OCRDs)
PANDAS	pediatric autoimmune neuropsychiatric disorder associated with streptococcal infection (PANDAS)
PD	Parkinson's disease (PD)
q-EEG	Quantitative analysis of the EEG (q-EEG)
QTLs	methylation quantitative trait loci (QTLs)
rTMS	repetitive transcranial magnetic stimulation (rTMS)
SN	substantia nigra (SN)
SNc	substantia nigra pars compacta (SNc)
SNPs	single nucleotide polymorphisms (SNPs)
SNr	substantia nigra pars reticulata (SNr)
SNRIs	Serotonin–Norepinephrine Reuptake Inhibitors (SNRIs)
SRIs	serotonin reuptake inhibitors (SRIs)
STN	subthalamic nucleus (STN)
TCA	tricyclic antidepressant (TCA)

TS   Tourette's Syndrome (TS)
VTA   ventral tegmental area (VTA)
Y-BOCS   Yale-Brown Obsessive Compulsive Scale (Y-BOCS)

INTRODUCTION

Obsessive-compulsive disorder (OCD) is a serious multifactorial psychiatric illness.

OCD has a lifetime prevalence of 2.5%, which increases when subthreshold obsessive-compulsive symptoms are considered. Due to its prevalence and associated comorbidities, it has been considered as one of the 10 major causes of disability, together with major depression, schizophrenia, bipolar disorder and alcoholism [1].

While inpatient admissions of OCD patients are uncommon, the elevated rates of comorbidity and higher admission rates are warning about the importance of patient screening for OCD and the need for outpatient treatment [2].

Furthermore, its centrality in a set of conditions defined in DSM V as obsessive-compulsive and related disorders (OCRDs) gives the disorder a prominent role in the wide and complex range of the psychiatric pathology [3].

OCD is characterized by specific symptoms and clinical manifestations, such as: distressing intrusive thoughts, obsessions, and task-oriented repetitive, time-consuming actions, compulsions, planned to contrast these intrusive thoughts and often to decrease the amount of anxiety. Typical compulsive behaviors include excessive handwashing, repetitive checking, and concern for order and symmetry. Typical obsessions are represented by concerns about contamination, morally unacceptable sexual or religious thoughts, safety or harm, unwanted acts of aggression, repetitive checking, and concern for order and symmetry.

The age of onset of OCD shows a bimodal pattern, with symptoms appearing during childhood/adolescence more frequently in males and in early adulthood in women. OCD often presents itself with comorbidities ranging from neurological, rheumatological and psychiatric diseases. The presence of another psychiatric disorder as a comorbidity during a lifetime is about 90% among individuals with OCD. Anxiety disorders (75.8%), mood disorders (63.3%) and impulse control disorders (ICD) (55.9%) are reported to be the most frequent comorbidities. Despite the growing acknowledgement in terms of distress associated with the disorder, thoughts or behaviors in patients with OCD have been underestimated. Recently, significantly higher rates of suicidal behaviors have been reported in OCD patients. Thus, suicide risk should be carefully monitored in these patients, particularly in those who have previously attempted suicide [4]. OCD is commonly assumed as being caused by multiple factors such as a combination of stress, genetic susceptibility, and interference with neurochemical substances. Therefore, OCD has been recognized as a heterogeneous, polygenic neuropsychiatric disorder [5].

In addition, neuroanatomical studies using fMri have revealed the anatomical basis of the disorder. Evidence that OCD responds selectively to serotonin reuptake inhibitors (SRIs) has led to a considerable emphasis on the serotonergic system [6].

Dopamine system involvement was highlighted after the response of patients to SRIs augmentation with dopamine D2 receptor antagonists or dopamine blockers. Indeed, many other systems play a role [7, 8].

However, there is also increasing evidence that a specific infantile type of OCD can be a self-immune disorder [9].

OCD can present a significant management challenge to the clinical psychiatrist. Individuals with OCD might not benefit from standard therapies both pharmacological (SSRIs-, or clomipramine) and psychosocial interventions, such as 40% of subjects with OCD do not have a "true" clinical response or gain little benefit from these treatment strategies; therefore, those are called treatment-resistant [10]. Augmentation strategies have been explored for patients refractory to proven interventions, but they are not as of yet robustly supported by controlled studies. The combination of medication with psychotherapy is often used, though careful studies have not documented synergistic benefit in adult patients. OCD refractory to available treatments remains a profound clinical challenge.

In this chapter we give an overview on OCD ranging from epidemiology, diagnosis, symptoms and comorbidities to neurochemistry, neuroanatomy, and treatment of this complex disease.

EPIDEMIOLOGY

OCD occurs worldwide, with common features across different ethnic groups and cultures [11].

Age of onset in OCD has a bimodal distribution trend in which almost 50% of all OCD cases are manifested [12, 13] with an early onset in childhood, and a late-onset adult expression. Early-onset OCD, with a mean age of 11 years, generally appears to be more severe, more familial, and more predominant in males. Furthermore, juvenile onset is related to tic- disorders, lack of therapeutic response and stronger genetic relations. It has also been described a pediatric autoimmune neuropsychiatric disorder associated with streptococcal infection (PANDAS) [14].

The adulthood expression has a mean age of 23 years. Males generally tend to have an earlier age of onset than females, but in adulthood females exceed males by a slight, resulting in a distribution between sex that is roughly the same. An onset after 40 years age is rare but in some patients this disorder starts later, for example, after pregnancy, miscarriage, or parturition [12, 13].

Individuals with OCD frequently have other psychiatric disorders concurrently or at some time in their lives [15] and a sub-classification of OCD based on comorbidity has been proposed [16]. A major question in the assessment of comorbidities is that treatment non-responsiveness frequently implies the presence of comorbid conditions. Unresponsive patients are more likely to meet criteria for comorbid conditions such as bipolar disorder (BD) and attention deficit hyperactivity disorder (ADHD).

Epidemiological studies frequently report a high degree of comorbidity between OCD and Tourette's syndrome/tic disorders, with prevalence estimates ranging from 26 to 59% [17].

SYMPTOMS AND CLINICAL MANIFESTATIONS

OCD is related to work and social impairment and to an important emotional impact [9]. Furthermore, OCD patients report worse quality of life than patients with heroin dependence or depressed patients. This is largely due to the disabling and pervasive nature of its symptoms: obsessions, distressing intrusive thoughts and task-oriented repetitive, time-consuming actions, compulsions, planned to contrast these thoughts and often decrease the amount of anxiety. It is interesting to observe that all main symptoms associated with OCD have been widely described from the past. The German psychiatrist Carl Westphal, who first made a definition of OCD in 1877, used the word "Zwangsvorstellung", coined by combining the German words "Zwang", constriction, and "Vorstellung", idea, describing the intrusiveness of thoughts that is characteristic of the disorder and the severity of the experience of those suffering from the condition.

Before 1877, OCD was mainly described in relation to religious or moral issues, reporting a mismatch between subjective goals and behavior. This perception was accompanied by preservation of insight about what often many patients define as bizarre behavior and is one of the most representative sides of the disorder. This discrepancy is so called "egodystonia" and is one of the many complexities that OCD presents to the clinician or neuroscientist [18].

Typical compulsive behaviors include excessive handwashing, repetitive checking, arranging rituals, counting, repeating routine activities, hoarding [19] and concern for order and symmetry. To deal with obsessions, patients try to ignore them, suppress them, or to counterbalance them with another thought or action. Typical obsessions are represented by concerns about contamination, morally unacceptable sexual or religious thoughts, safety or harm, unwanted acts of aggression, repetitive checking, and concern for order and symmetry. In response to an obsession or to reduce distress, compulsions are performed.

Several studies over the last decade tried to investigate the variance of OCD symptom clusters in different OCD patient populations through factors and clusters analysis or latent variables of symptom inventories. The majority found support the evidence of three to five symptoms dimensions [20].

The most commonly identified symptoms patterns include four dimensions: 1- contamination obsessions and cleaning compulsions; 2- aggressive, sexual, religious, and somatic obsessions with control-related compulsions; 3- obsessions regarding symmetry, exactness, and the need for things to be "right" coupled with compulsions related to ordering, arranging, and counting; and 4- accumulation obsessions and compulsions (Table 1).

Table 1. OCD symptom dimension

Obsessions	Compulsions
• Fear of germs or contamination	• Checking
• Repugnant thoughts	• Washing or cleaning
• Fear of causing harm accidently or intentionally towards others or self	• Repetitive thoughts
	• Repeatedly behaviors
• Order and symmetry	• Excessive rereading or rewriting
• Religious and moral believes	• Ordering or arranging
• Intrusive sexual thoughts	
• Images of violent scenes	

Furthermore, sensory phenomena, premonitory impulses and "right" perceptions whereby the patient continues his compulsions until there is a feeling that things are "right" and they can stop, may also be present in OCD [21].

When describing symptoms, it is also useful to consider the numerous comorbidities that characterize the disorder that may influence its clinical features. For instance, when the disorder is comorbid with tics, it is characterized by high awareness. While when in comorbidity with mood disorders it presents features of obsessive-compulsive personality disorder, high score on the "taboo" factor of OCD symptoms, and low consciousness [22].

DIAGNOSIS AND CLASSIFICATION

The diagnosis of OCD symptoms is frequently challenging, and management requires a unique approach, with specific adaptations in pharmacologic and psychotherapeutic treatments when compared to mood or other anxiety disorders. It has been suggested that only 14% to 56% of patients seek treatment, and recognition and diagnosis is typically delayed by 8 to 10 years.

Table 2. Obsessive-compulsive-related disorders, as proposed for DSM-5

- Obsessive-compulsive disorder
- Obsessive-compulsive personality disorder
- Tourette's syndrome
- Grooming disorders
    - Trichotillomania
    - Excoriation (skin picking)
    - Nail biting
- Body dysmorphic disorder
- Eating disorders

With the advent of DSM V OCD moved out from the category of "anxiety disorders" and is placed in an autonomous category defined "Obsessive-Compulsive and Related Disorders (OCRDs) with body dysmorphic disorder (BDD), trichotillomania (TTM; hair-pulling disorder), excoriation (skin-picking) disorder, hoarding disorder, substance/medication-induced OCRD, OCRD due to another medical condition, and other specified OCRDs [23] (Table 2).

While OCD shares many characteristics with related anxiety disorders, the shift of OCD to OCRDs was motivated by the fact that not all patients suffering from OCD experience anxiety, evidence that suggests that is not the central component of OCD and related disorders, rather a secondary manifestation. Those suggestions were confirmed by neuroimaging, phenotypical, and genetic and response to treatment [24-26]. Although they belong to the same category, the differentiation between OCD and other related disorders is substantial and is based on precise differences in the contents and the character of the thought and behavioral processes.

The DSM-V diagnostic criteria for OCD are represented by the presence of obsessions, compulsions, or both:

- Obsessions are defined by the following:
  - Recurrent and persistent thoughts, urges, or impulses that are experienced, at some time during the disturbance, as intrusive and unwanted, and that in most individuals cause marked anxiety or distress.
  - The individual attempts to ignore or suppress such thoughts, urges, or images, or to neutralize them with some other thought or action (that is, by performing a compulsion).
- Compulsions are defined by the following:
  - Repetitive behaviors (for example, hand washing, ordering or checking) or mental acts (for example, praying, counting or repeating words silently) that the individual feels driven to perform in response to an obsession or according to rules that must be applied rigidly.
  - The behaviors or mental acts are aimed at preventing or reducing anxiety or distress, or preventing some dreaded event or situation; however, these behaviors or mental acts are not connected in a realistic way with what they are designed to neutralize, or prevent, or are clearly excessive.

The obsessions or compulsions are time-consuming (for example take >1 hour per day) or cause clinically significant distress or impairment in social, occupational, or other important areas of functioning.

The obsessive–compulsive symptoms are not attributable to the physiological effects of a substance (for example, a drug of abuse or a medication) or another medical condition.

Specify if:

- With good or fair insight: the individual recognizes that OCD beliefs are definitely or probably not true or that they may or may not be true
- With poor insight: the individual thinks OCD beliefs are probably true
- With absent insight/delusional beliefs: the individual is completely convinced that OCD beliefs are true

Specify if:

- Tic-related: the individual has a current or past history of a tic disorder

The addition of a tic specifier to DSM-V reflects the unique difference between individuals with tics in comorbidity and those without, particularly in relation to response to drug treatment, which appears to be influenced by the presence of tics [27, 28].

Young children may not be able to articulate the aims of these behaviors or mental acts [29].

Valid screening tools for the primary care setting are therefore essential in the clinical routine. These include the semi-structured, clinically administered Yale-Brown Obsessive Compulsive Scale (Y-BOCS) [30] [19] is considered the gold standard for assessing the symptoms and severity of OCD. The Y-BOCS assesses the presence of 64 obsessions and compulsions as well as the severity of associated symptoms. Several short forms of self-assessment are available, an example of which is the Obsessive-Compulsive Inventory, Short Version (OCI-SV) [31].

The Obsessive-Compulsive Inventory, which typically takes 5 minutes to complete, demonstrates moderate convergence with the Y-BOCS, and consists of 18 items (each rated from 0 to 4, depending on the degree of associated distress). Scores greater than or equal to 21 (out of 72) on the OCI-SV suggest the presence of OCD.

Quantitative analysis of the EEG (q-EEG) in patients with OCD showed a decreased beta and an increased theta power at frontotemporal regions. At least two subtypes of qEEG OCD patients within a clinically homogeneous group of patients who met DSM-III-R criteria for OCD were recognized. 80.0% of the members of subtype 1 were found to be non-responders to drug treatment, while 82.4% of the members of subtype 2 were found to be treatment responders [32, 33].

Due to the heterogeneity of OCD neurobiology, assessing the quantitative EEG of OCD patients could be useful before deciding about treatment strategy and for predicting treatment response [34].

DIFFERENTIAL DIAGNOSIS

Approaching the diagnosis, it is crucial to make a differentiation between OCD and other psychiatric disorders that may enter into differential diagnosis with it. It is important to distinguish between these conditions because there are significant differences in terms of treatment approach. In BDD, the focus is exclusively on perceived defects in the individual's appearance. Hoarding disorder concerns exclusively the difficulty in discarding and the accumulation of objects that results. In trichotillomania and excoriation disorders, the focus is on repetitive hair pulling or skin picking, respectively, and is not accompanied by triggering obsessions. Patients with an anxiety disorder may report recurrent thoughts or worries, typically related to real life. Individuals with a generalized anxiety disorder may express excessive worries about losing their job or about the health and well-being of their family members. In social phobia, exaggerated worries are notable but related to the possibility of embarrassing oneself in social interactions. Depressed individuals may express ruminations that are typically mood correlated and not experienced as intrusive, which differentiates them from obsessions.

Other frequent differential psychiatric diagnoses include:

- Eating disorders, where the main concerns are focused on food, weight or body image.
- Illness anxiety disorder, which is characterized by recurrent thoughts related to the fear of having a serious illness. In contrast, in individuals with somatic obsessions, the worry is typically of contracting the disease in the future, and other obsessive content will also be present. Tic disorders are characterized by sudden, rapid, recurrent and non-rhythmic behavior not triggered by obsessions.
- Psychotic disorders presenting with hallucinations or formal thought disorders, differ from OCD patients with poor insight or OCD patients who may be delusional with regard to obsessions.
- Obsessive-compulsive personality disorder, which, despite its similarity in name, is not directly related to OCD. It is characterized by a long-standing pattern of perfectionism and rigidity, but will be perceived by the individual as appropriate, rather than reported as intrusive in the way the obsessions are experienced. These individuals will not have frank obsessions or compulsions [35].

COMORBIDITY

Psychiatric Comorbidity

Unresponsive patients to treatment often present comorbid conditions. Particularly, comorbid conditions such as BD and ADHD are common in treatment-resistant patients, but only few studies have investigated their impact on treatment resistance [36].

The strong association between OCD and affective disorders is well documented [37, 38].

Depression is the most frequent complication of OCD, as reported in several studies [39]. One-third of patients with OCD have concurrent Major Depression Disorder (MDD) at the time of evaluation. MDD was 10 times more prevalent in OCD patients than in the general population and up to 60–80% of patients with OCD experience a depressive episode in their lifetime, one-third of patients with OCD have concurrent MDD at the time of evaluation [40, 41].

BD comorbidity in OCD is a relevant phenomenon and has clinically significant influence on the symptomatologic expression and complications of the disorder [42]. Moreover, comorbidity with BD has relevant implications for treatment outcome, since bipolarity has a negative influence on compliance and response to currently available anti-obsessive agents [43, 44].

Clinical and epidemiological studies have suggested that the rate of lifetime comorbid BD in clinical and epidemiological samples of patients with OCD is up to 21.5% [40, 45]. In advance almost 50% of OCD cases manifest cyclothymic traits and/or some lifetime hypomanic symptoms [44]. Bipolar subjects with OCD were more likely than those without OCD to have higher lifetime rates of thoughts of death and suicide and of suicide attempts [46].

Patients with OCD have classically been considered at low risk for suicide, with reports of completed suicides in less than 1% [59] and history of suicide attempts in 3–4% of samples [60]. Nonfatal suicidal behavior occurs in nearly 15% of individuals suffering from OCD [61].

ADHD is a common childhood-onset neurodevelopmental disorder that occurs in approximately 5% of the population, which frequently co-occurs with OCD [53]. Family studies suggest that OCD and ADHD may co-segregate in families [54].

Post-streptococcal autoimmunity is hypothesized to be an additional etiologic pathway in a subset of children with OCD and tic disorders

[55]. This subset of children experiences a sudden onset of OCD and/or motor tics in association with Group A streptococcal (GAS) infections (e.g., "strep throat"), a disorder classified as pediatric autoimmune neuropsychiatric disorders associated with streptococcal infections (PANDAS).

The prevalence of comorbid OCD and schizophrenia was estimated at 12.2% by the US National Institute for Mental Health Epidemiologic Catchment Area Study [47].

There is growing evidence that patients with comorbid OCD and schizophrenia (recently termed "schizo-obsessive") [48] appear to have distinct patterns of psychopathology, course of illness, psychiatric comorbidity, neurocognitive deficits, and treatment response, compared to their schizophrenic counterparts, suggesting the existence of a separate subgroup on the schizophrenia spectrum [49].

Neurological Comorbidity

Even if the association between OCD and Parkinson disease (PD) is controversial, recent evidences highlighted higher incidence of OCD in PD, that would further strengthen the hypothesized involvement of fronto-basal ganglia circuitry in the manifestation of OCD [50].

Roughly one-third to one-half of children with Tourette syndrome (TS) or chronic tic disorder will experience comorbid OCD throughout their lifetime [51]. OCD symptoms in patients with TS have an onset around the time that the tics reach their *worst-ever*, but symptoms may also appear *de novo* in adulthood. OCD patients with comorbid tics tend to have greater rates of symmetry obsessions, and counting, repeating, ordering, and arranging compulsions than OCD patients without comorbid tic symptoms [52].

OCD is frequently described in patients with primarily basal ganglia dysfunction, such as TS, Sydenham's chorea, Huntington's disease, and von Economo's encephalitis [53].

Immunological and Inflammatory Comorbidities

A growing body of evidence highlights the involvement of autoimmune mechanisms in the pathophysiology of a subset of OCD [54]. There is a strong correlation between OCD and different inflammatory markers, as well as rheumatological biomarkers. These correlations have been demonstrated in both adult and pediatric populations [55].

There is a higher incidence of subsequent OCD among patients with systemic autoimmune diseases (SADs). Specifically, the risk of OCD was observed to be significant increase in systemic lupus erythematosus, dermatomyositis, and Sjögren's syndrome [56]. Multiple inflammatory and rheumatological markers have been studied among patients with OCD and some studies reported that tumor necrosis factor-alpha (TNF-α) marker was found elevated in these patients [57].

Other Comorbidities

Finally, experts assume that a flare-up of symptoms linked to Covid-19 particularly affects people with OCD, particularly those with washing compulsions [58]. Perhaps no group of individuals with mental illness is as directly affected by the worsening outbreak of COVID-19 as people living with OCD. For these people, coronavirus can become all they think about [59].

NEUROANATOMY

In this section the three systems involved will be briefly described: basal ganglia, the motor loop and the limbic system, cognitive/associative loop.

The basal ganglia are a set of subcortical nuclei whose main function is to control movement. Since the basal ganglia in addition to the motor component have a limbic and associative component, these are also involved in the mechanisms that regulate behavior, emotions, executive functions and motor learning. The primary structures of the basal ganglia are known as striatum (caudate and putamen) and globus pallidus. Additional structures important for the function of the basal ganglia are the subthalamic nucleus (STN) located in the diencephalon, the substantia nigra (SN) located in the midbrain and the pedunculopontine nucleus in the pons [60, 61].

The motor loop is the most studied of the three loops. The motor loop has three pathways, the direct which facilitates movement, and the indirect and hyperdirect which inhibit movement. The striatum receives glutamatergic input from the cerebral cortex and modulating dopaminergic input from the substantia nigra *pars compacta* (SNc). The input from SNc can be both excitatory (direct pathway) or inhibitory (indirect pathway) depending on which receptor in the striatum that receives the input. The dopamine receptor type mostly found in neurons of the direct pathway is called D1, and for the indirect pathway, it is called D2. In the direct pathway, the striatum sends GABAergic projections to the substantia nigra *pars reticulata* (SNr) and internal globus pallidus (GPi). The inhibition of these two basal ganglia output structures results in disinhibition of ventro-lateral thalamus. When the thalamus no longer is inhibited, it can facilitate movement. Because neurotransmission from the GPi and SNr is tonic, this means that ventro-lateral thalamus is inhibited in the absence of input from the direct pathway. This inhibition of the thalamus needs to be overcome to initiate movement by activation of the motor cortex. In the indirect pathway, the striatum inhibits the external globus pallidus (GPe) via GABAergic projections, which result in disinhibition of the STN. The STN is a glutamatergic structure, and its disinhibition leads to excitation of the SNr and GPi. The hyperdirect pathway instead works by excitatory projections directly from the cerebral cortex to the STN, and has the same effect as the indirect pathway [62] (Figure 1).

> DIRECT PATHWAY: Orbito-frontal cortex → Ventromedial Caudate → Globus pallidus and Substantia Nigra → Mediodorsal Thalamus
> INDIRECT PATHWAY: Orbito-frontal cortex → Ventromedial Caudate → Indirect Basal Ganglial Control System → Globus Pallidus and Substantia Nigra → Mediodorsal Thalamus

Figure 1. Direct and indirect pathways of the orbito-subcortical circuit connecting neuroanatomical structures hypothesised to be associated with symptoms.

Concerning the *limbic loop*, structures similar to those of the motor loop are involved. For example, nucleus accumbens ((NAc) part of the striatum), is active in the limbic loop. The dopaminergic input comes from the ventral tegmental area (VTA) instead of the Nc, while the GABAergic input comes from the ventral pale instead of the pale globe. Furthermore, the part of the STN that affects the limbic loop is more ventro-medial than the motor loop, and is called the limbic tip of the STN. The exit structures project to the mid-dorsal rather than ventro-lateral thalamus which is more typical for the motor loop. The limbic functions of STN are important for reward and motivation [62, 63].

The *cognitive/associative loop* has been shown to be important for direct behaviors, decision making and attention. Furthermore, impulsivity is a feature of this cycle. This circuit receives projections from the cerebral cortex to the anterior caudate in the striatum. The anterior caudate then projects via GABAergic neurons to the GPi and SNr, and these in turn inhibit the anterior dorsal and ventral nuclei of the thalamus [62, 63].

Despite the large amount of published studies about OCD and the high prevalence of the disease, the underlying pathogenesis of OCD is not yet fully known. Clinical observations, together with evidences showing the association between OC symptoms, post- encephalitis parkinsonian and striatal lesions, suggested that specific neuronal circuits are involved and mediate the pathogenesis of the disease. Neuroimaging studies have helped to confirm that abnormalities in core brain regions are involved in the pathophysiology of OCD [64, 65, 66]. In fact, these abnormalities are consistent with cortico-striatal-thalamic-cortical dysfunction (CSTC) and impaired inhibition, and evidence suggests that they are specific to OCD [67].

OCD symptoms are well documented in various neurological disorders with striatal involvement, including TS, Sydenham's chorea, Huntington's disorder, and PD. Particularly, the orbito-fronto-striato-thalamo-cortical circuit involving the basal ganglia appears to be damaged in OCD. The greater activation of the left orbitofrontal cortex and of the bilateral caudate nucleus is associated with an overestimation of the negative consequences of a certain action, which would be at the basis of obsessive thoughts. The increase in the activity of the anterior cingulate cortex favors a greater interpretation of the verifiability of negative consequences associated with an anxious response, underlying the activation of the limbic system. Lesions of the globus pallidus (by virtue of the resulting thalamic disinhibition) have also been associated with OCD [68].

The neurons in the STN behave differently in people with OCD: STN neurons in patients with OCD tend to fire at a lower rate and display a bursting pattern. In OCD the bursts are more common in the STN in the left hemisphere [69].

Disturbances in the brain's reward network also underline OCD. Not surprisingly, the ventral capsule/ventral striatum and the NAc region are a clinically approved target for deep brain stimulation for OCD [70].

A large proportion of neuroimaging studies have found abnormalities in precuneus structure and function in OCD population. Precuneus is an important functional hub of the brain in the default mode network (DMN) for the integration of internally and externally guided information. Furthermore, a reduced grey matter volume, an increased cortical thickness and an increased white matter volume in precuneus, were reported in OCD patients. An increased activation of the precuneus under neutral emotional stimulation has been related to the severity of the patient's obsessive-compulsive symptoms. Emerging evidence demonstrated that also the cerebellar networks were tightly involved in cognitive processing in psychiatric disorders [71, 72].

NEUROCHEMISTRY

Several neurotransmitter systems are involved in the pathogenesis of OCD, including: serotoninergic system, dopaminergic system and glutamatergic system, highlighting the importance of neurotransmitters in sustaining OCD symptoms. Many studies have been focused on abnormalities in the cortico-striatal-thalamic-cortical (CSTC) loop pathways, so that nowadays the treatment targets are DA and 5-HT systems. Even though some studies highlight the role of serotoninergic system in OCD pathogenesis, there is not a strong evidence yet about an underlying serotonin deficiency playing a primary causal role in OCD [73].

Treatments with SRIs and the consequent neuroendocrine response have raised questions about the role of specific serotoninergic receptors (5-HT) involved in the etiopathogenesis of OCD. For instance, the effects of mCPP on the postsynaptic 5-HT2C receptor could be particularly relevant [74, 75]. Data also suggest a role for the terminal autoreceptor 5-HT1D, desensitization of this receptor in the orbitofrontal cortex requires the administration of high-dose, long-lasting SRIs [76]. Data also support a role for 5-HT1D in OCD.

However, although the role of serotonin system in mediating OCD is remarkable, so far no specific abnormality in serotonin system has been identified as a cause. Indeed, many other systems, including glutamate neurotransmission, gonadal steroid neuropeptides also play a role and the role of second and third messenger pathways in OCD needs to be delineated [7, 8].

Involvement of dopaminergic systems is evidenced after patients respond to increased SRIs with dopamine D2 receptor antagonists. Dopamine blockers are used in the treatment of TS, one of the spectrum of OCD. To substantiate the contribution of dopamine to OCD, some studies have reported an association between variants in catecholaminergic genes (including COMT) and OCD [77, 78], and molecular imaging studies have demonstrated alterations in specific dopaminergic receptors, such as a decrease in striatal dopamine D2 receptors, in OCD [79, 80].

Neurochemical and genetic evidences suggest also a glutamate dysregulation in OCD, although much remains still unclear [81]. One of the most direct evidence for abnormalities in glutamate comes from the examination of cerebrospinal fluid (CSF), that contains elevated glutamate levels, although it's still not known whether it comes from (an abnormality or a reflection of disruption in a specific brain circuit) [82, 83]. Other authors evidenced abnormalities in a glutamate transporter (EAAT3), which might reduce clearance and so grow glutamate levels in CSF [84], and in the glutamate receptor gene GRIK2 and PTPRD, which are involved in the development of glutamatergic synapses [85].

Neurogenetics

Many works suggest that OCD has a family component. Studies have shown a genetic relationship between OCD and other disorders such as anorexia, TS, and ADHD [86].

The first GWAS of 1,465 early-onset cases found no single nucleotide polymorphisms (SNPs) that achieved genome-wide significance, but there was an implication of methylation quantitative trait loci (QTLs) and frontal lobe expression (e) QTLs [87].

Regarding the serotonergic system, studies have confirmed that 5-HT1D polymorphism, plays an important role in mediating OCD [88].

Concerning dopaminergic polymorphisms, it has emerged that that alleles were distributed differently in patients with OCD with and without tics [89].

About the glutamate system, emerged the evidence of modal impairment of cortical-striatal function and possible glutamate-GABA imbalance in OCD in these circuits [90].

To sum up, the most recent evidences confirm that OCD is etiologically multifactorial and it involves several groups of genes. A future perspective should be a better understanding of the phenotypic and therapeutic heterogeneity, in order to obtain personalized treatments.

TREATMENT

According to the National Institute for Health and Care Excellence (NICE) [91] CG31 guidelines first-line treatments for OCD patients with mild functional impairment should be represented by cognitive-behavioral therapy (CBT) and exposure/response prevention (ERP)[92, 93]. In case these treatments result ineffective, SRIs medications and more intensive cycles of CBT must be considered [94, 95]. Unfortunately, approximately 25%–40% of patients fails to respond to either modality and few patients experience complete symptoms resolution [96]. If treatment response is not adequate and no side effects have occurred after 4-6 weeks, SRIs dosage increases may be considered. Higher dosages have shown better efficacy [97], although lower doses could be effective in preventing relapses [98]. When SRIs and CBT integrated therapy fail, the only medication approach with substantial empirical support is the use of antipsychotics as augmentation. This approach has been demonstrated even more useful for patients with a comorbid chronic tic disorder [99]. After symptoms remission, treatment should be carried on for no less than 12 months, in order to prevent further relapse. Moreover, the number of previous episodes, the presence of residual symptoms and concomitant psychosocial impairment might be considered to evaluate a further prolongation of treatment [91].

However, only a few studies have addressed the issue of how long to continue pharmacotherapy, once a clinical response has been achieved. This is, of course, a complex decision in individual cases, with benefit being weighed in the context of side effects, patient attitudes, comorbidities, the potential for drug interactions, pregnancy and lactation, and other factors. OCD is often a chronic condition, and remission is unfortunately rare. Treatment of an episode to remission followed by treatment discontinuation is, therefore, not a common clinical scenario [94].

Unfortunately, the relapse rates in individuals switched from stable active pharmacotherapy to placebo approximately are double those in patients maintained on their SRIs pharmacotherapy. In general, once symptom improvement on a stable medication regimen has been achieved, these results suggest that continuation of treatment is advisable, in the absence of intolerable side effects or other case-specific factors [100]. Therefore, a long term OCD pharmacological management is often necessary.

Nevertheless, even with an optimal pharmacological treatment, many patients continue to experience significant symptoms. Therefore, the need for new treatment strategies is an urgent issue. The therapeutic use of nutraceutics in augmentation among individuals with refractory- OCD to the first- line pharmacological interventions, or in monotherapy, represents a potential alternative in OCD treatment.

The evidence for an increased activity in brain regions that form a cortico-striato-thalamo-cortical (CSTC) loop in OCD patients paved the way for anatomically targeted treatments as neuromodulation with either noninvasive devices (e.g., transcranial magnetic stimulation, TMS) or invasive procedures (e.g., deep brain stimulation, DBS) [101].

Here we review evidence-based pharmacotherapies for OCD, as well as alternatives that may be considered in refractory patients.

PHARMACOTHERAPY

Selective Serotonin Reuptake Inhibitors (SSRIs)

The interest in the role of serotonin in OC disorder sparked in 1975 by the observation of clomipramine beneficial role in OCD treatment. Selective SRIs (SSRIs), such as fluvoxamine and sertraline, has shown to be more effective than placebo without significant differences between them [102] and they have been established as the mainstay for pharmacological management of OCD.

Several studies have been conducted starting from early 1980s investigating the role of the serotonin system in OCD, but findings were either equivocal or conflicting and randomized controlled trials failed to confirm the efficacy of augmentation with serotonergic agents [103-105] and antidepressants that do not bind with high affinity to the serotonin transporter are generally ineffective for OCD.

One of the most accredited hypotheses of SRIs efficacy sees SRIs work restoring balance between direct and indirect frontal-cortical pathways [106] and operate on orbitofrontal-subcortical circuits that drive OC behavior.

Major positive factors with SSRI treatment efficacy are family history for OCD, aggressive, sexual, and religious obsessions, orbitofrontal cortex hypometabolism and right caudate nucleus hypermetabolism [107, 108], meanwhile hoarding behavior and poor insight correlated with limited SSRI treatment response.

SSRIs are more efficacious in OCD when used at high doses, in excess of the typical dose range established by their suppliers (which are generally derived from studies of MDD. OCD symptoms typically also take longer to respond to SSRIs monotherapy than do those of MDD; an adequate trial is 8–12 weeks [93]. The reasons for these differences between OCD and MDD response to SSRIs remain unclear.

Paroxetine doses of 40-60 mg/day are correlated with significant symptom improvement and decrease the rate of relapse in OCD patients. Nevertheless, some authors have reached dosages up to 100 mg/day to see clinically meaningful improvements [93]. Paroxetine showed a marked anxiolytic effect and may be recommended as a first-line therapy in the treatment of OCD comorbidities [109].

Fluvoxamine (dosage range 100-300 mg/day) showed efficacy in social anxiety, avoidance, and phobic symptoms after 6-8 weeks of treatment [110]. Caution must be used when the patient is treated in polypharmacy. Indeed, Fluvoxamine is a potent inhibitor of the liver enzyme CYP2C19 and thus inhibits the metabolism of other drugs. This can result in marked elevations of serum levels of the other drug when the two agents are co-administered, raising the risk of side effects [111].

Citalopram is effective at doses of 20-60 mg/day [112], with improvements on psychosocial functioning, depressive symptoms, obsessive thoughts, repetitive behaviour, and anxiety. Although it has a good tolerability profile, doses above 20 mg/day are not recommended in the elderly, and it is recommended that the drug be avoided altogether in individuals with a QTc of greater than 500 msec or with conditions that predispose to arrhythmia [113]. This complicates the clinical use of citalopram at high doses for OCD, and many clinicians have switched to escitalopram or another SSRI as an alternative. However, in patients who have clearly benefited from citalopram and do not wish to make a switch, ECG monitoring is advisable.

Escitalopram is the most 5-HT-selective among SSRIs and at the dosage of 20 mg/day (up to 40 mg/day according to some authors) is associated with an increase in response rate. Escitalopram is well tolerated and effective for long-term treatment and relapse prevention in OCD [98].

Fluoxetine is safe and effective at a dose of 40-60 mg/day, although some authors suggest increasing up to 80 mg/day [93] [114]. The effect of fluoxetine is particularly evident in the improvement of obsessive thoughts, washing compulsions, psychosocial functioning, and quality of life [115].

Sertraline shows efficacy and safety at doses of 50-200 mg/day, with a greater reduction in symptoms related to anxiety/fear, physical symptoms and avoidance behaviours [116]. Treatment of refractory OCD with high doses of sertraline (250-400 mg/day) resulted in a significant symptom improvement and a similar rate of adverse events observed with a 200 mg/day dose [117].

Clomipramine

Clomipramine is a tricyclic antidepressant (TCA) and was the first drug used to treat OCD because of his unique anti-obsessive effect due to its potent inhibition of serotonin reuptake. The efficacy of clomipramine in OCD, at a dosage of 200-250 mg/die, is equivalent to or slightly better than SSRIs, although its side effect profile is less favourable [118]. However, intravenous clomipramine is a possible strategy in treating refractory OCD [119].

In contrast to SSRIs, clomipramine has significant anticholinergic side effects (e.g., dry mouth and constipation), anti-histaminergic effects (e.g., weight gain and sedation) and alpha-adrenergic blocking effects (e.g., hypotension). It also has substantial arrhythmogenic potential; doses at or above the upper limit of the recommended dosing range, 250 mg, may require ECG monitoring, and cardiotoxicity in overdose is a concern. Clomipramine also carries a risk of seizure at doses above 250 mg. For all of these reasons, clomipramine is not generally considered a first-line agent. It remains an important alternative when SSRI monotherapy fails [93].

Serotonin–Norepinephrine Reuptake Inhibitors (SNRIs)

SNRIs combine the actions of SSRIs with inhibition of noradrenaline reuptake.

Venlafaxine shows satisfactory response rates with daily dosages between 150 mg/day and 375 mg/die [120]. It could be a good choice for patients with OCD that have not responded to prior SSRIs trials. Besides, his mechanism of action is similar to that of clomipramine, without exhibiting the problematic adverse effects related to histaminic, muscarinic, or adrenergic receptors block [121]. Venlafaxine is well tolerated, one concern regarding the long-term use has been the emergence of hypertension [122].

Duloxetine has shown some efficacy at high dosage in the treatment of OCD, although most evidence comes from case reports or studies with small samples [123].

While there continues to be some theoretical rationale for the use of SNRIs, these cannot be recommended for OCD monotherapy on the basis of currently available data [94].

Refractory OCD

A management strategy for treatment of refractory OCD patients consists of adding SSRIs to other drugs. Some open studies suggested that the combined treatment with clomipramine and an SSRI is effective and well tolerated, particularly in addition with citalopram [124], fluoxetine or sertraline [125]. An even faster response is possible with the intravenous administration of clomipramine or citalopram, but eventually, with continued treatment, the result is similar to oral administration [126].

Another important augmentation strategy is the use of antipsychotic drugs in add-on to SSRIs. According to the American Psychiatric Association guidelines, in cases of partial initial treatment response, the addition of low dosages of antipsychotics should be preferred over the switch to a different SSRI, which should be conducted only in case of non-response [93]. Despite no antipsychotic agent is officially approved for the treatment of OCD, about a third of patients were benefiting from the augmentation strategy with average antipsychotic doses.

In general, antipsychotic augmentation should not be considered until two SSRI trials of adequate dose and duration have been attempted, because of the more benign side effect profile of the SRIs and the reasonable likelihood of response to extended treatment or a switch to a second agent.

Risperidone was confirmed as a potential first choice at a dosage of 1-3 mg/die. Others possible adjuvant alternatives are haloperidol, quetiapine, olanzapine and aripiprazole [127].

Finally, augmentation with antiepileptic drugs it is a strategy to consider for a proportion of drug-resistant OCD patients. Add-on topiramate at daily dose ranges up to 400 mg improved refractory OCD [128]. Other associations are reported just in case reports or small group studies: Lamotrigine at 100-200 mg/day added on clomipramine or paroxetine obtained improvement [129, 130]; topiramate augmentation has been studied in treatment-refractory OCD patients with comorbid depression [131]; the addition of gabapentin to fluoxetine reduced time to treatment response [132].

Glutamatergic Agents: The NMDA Receptor

Glutamate transmission abnormalities in CSTC may contribute to the pathophysiology of OCD [94]. Consequentially, there is increasing interest in the use of glutamate-modulating agents in add-on or in monotherapy in refractory OCD.

Memantine acts as a noncompetitive NMDA receptor antagonist approved for the treatment of Alzheimer's disease. Recent studies show positive results in using memantine in treatment-resistant OCD in monotherapy at a dosage of 10-20 mg/die or in addition to fluvoxamine [133, 134] or in association with CBT. Side effects most commonly include fatigue, headache, increase in blood pressure and dizziness.

Ketamine is an open-channel nonselective antagonist at NMDA receptor. A cross-over RCT examined the effect of ketamine (0.5 mg/kg) intravenous infusion compared to saline infusion in medication-naïve patients with OCD [135]. Those receiving ketamine reported significant improvement in obsessions and the effect can persist for at last 1 week. The rapidity of onset of effects makes ketamine an attractive strategy but more researches are needed to explore the evidence.

Rilozule reduces glutamate outflow in cortical neurons and potentiate reuptake of extracellular glutamate by the glial cells [136]. In literature, it is reported modest benefits of riluzole augmentation in patients with refractory OCD [137].

N-acetyl cysteine (NAC) is the antioxidant precursor of glutathione (GSH), used to treat paracetamol poising or as a mucolytic in the treatment of airway diseases. Recently, studies have investigated the NAC effects on psychiatric conditions by virtue of its antioxidant properties. Specifically, NAC, acting in a double manner as a glutamate-modulating agent and as modulator of inflammatory pathways, has been used in OCD patients. Although NAC is easily accessible and has an optimal safety and tolerability profile, clinical studies regarding its effects on OCD symptoms are limited [138, 139]. However, NAC and nutraceutics in general should be considered when treating special populations such as young population and elders.

OTHER MEDICATIONS

Due to the high rate of treatment resistance and the significant disability in OCD patients, further clinical studies are needed to provide new treatment strategies. Promising results come from placebo-controlled studies concerning the efficacy of Ondansetron (5-HT3 antagonist) in monotherapy and in add on with SSRIs [140]; buprenorphine added on SSRIs or clomipramine [141]; D-cycloserine added on CBT [142] and cannabidiol [143].

Psychotherapy

CBT represents the first-line psychotherapy for OCD and different studies demonstrated that it significantly improves OCD symptoms both in adults and children [144]. In particular, CBT is based on the application of techniques of cognitive reappraisal and behavioural intervention.

Specifically, ERP (exposure and response prevention) is the treatment of choice for OCD. The patient is asked to involve gradual and prolonged exposure to fear-provoking stimuli, with or without the aid of relaxation techniques, combined with instructions to abstain from the compulsive behaviour. Eventually, the integration of ERP with cognitive components is important to help the patient to identify, modify and stop the automatic thoughts related to obsessions [145].

CBT (ERP with cognitive reappraisal) can be delivered in individual or group, in-person or by internet-based protocols [146]. Besides, protocols of intensive CBT (multiple sessions over a few days) for OCD have been tested for severe, treatment-resistant patients and as a first-line treatment [147].

Deep TMS for Treatment-Resistant OCD

In the last few years, several studies have been conducted investigating OCD treating with repetitive transcranial magnetic stimulation (rTMS) [148]. However, so far, a unique protocol has not been identified relatively to stimulation target, frequency, and intensity, and different stimulation sites have yielded contradictory findings. A recent meta-analysis [149] found active rTMS to be clinically and statistically superior to sham treatment [150] and the Food and Drug Administration (FDA) approved the deep TMS (dTMS) for the treatment of OCD.

OCD involves functional and anatomical abnormalities with an hyperactivation of CSTC, the orbitofrontal cortex (OFC), the anterior cingulate cortex (ACC), and ventral striatum [151]. These structures hyperactivation decrease after successful treatments [152]. Precisely, the ACC is involved in processes that are impaired in OCD patients, including integration of thoughts, response selection before a movement occurs, error monitoring and the detection of cognitive conflicts [153].

High-frequency dTMS over the ACC significantly improved OCD symptoms and may be considered as a potential intervention for patients who do not respond adequately to pharmacological and psychological interventions. Moreover, initial trials indicate that dTMS stimulation is safe and effective and no severe adverse events occurred, except for mild headache during or immediately after stimulation [101].

Neurosurgery

For the most severe and refractory cases, neurosurgical interventions must be taken into account. These treatments are performed in a specific region, but their influence spreads to include the larger dysfunctional network.

Stereotactic Ablation

The two most common ablation procedures are dorsal anterior cingulotomy [154] and anterior capsulotomy [155] and they interrupt pathways in CSTC circuits reducing their hyperactivation.

Deep Brain Stimulation

Firstly used to treat patients with movement disorders such as PD and essential tremor, the Deep Brain Stimulation (DBS) may represent an alternative novel treatment, which can modulate neuronal excitability, activity, and plasticity. It has the advantages of being explantable and adjustable [156]. The FDA approved a Humanitarian Device Exemption for Ventral Capsule/Ventral Striatum DBS in intractable OCD based upon the device's safety record and evidence of benefit for cases of severe and treatment refractory OCD [156]. Unfortunately, because of the expensive costs and challenges in manage this therapy, the number of DBS for OCD procedures are still very few.

CONCLUSION

In the wide and complex range of psychiatric disorders, OCD has been recognized as one of the most disabling psychiatric illnesses. Obsessions and the associated bizarre ritualistic behavioral patterns can lead to significant impairments in personal, social, and occupational function for OCD patients. In fact, depression, suicidality, functional impairment and days housebound are often associated to OCD. OCD can present a significant management challenge to the clinical psychiatrist. Different OCD subtypes have been hypothesized which may account for different response to therapy and different pathophysiological mechanisms. Despite significant therapeutic advances, there remain several challenges in treating OCD. Integrated understanding of the pathophysiology of OCD in the context of dimensional psychiatry and future directions for research are discussed in the chapter.

REFERENCES

[1] (WHO), W.H.O., *The 'Newly Defined' Burden of Mental Problems.* 1999.

[2] Brakoulias, V. and G. Sara, Hospital admissions for obsessive-compulsive disorder in NSW, 1997 to 2010. *Australas Psychiatry,* 2011. 19(6): p. 502-6.

[3] American Psychiatric Association, *Diagnostic and Statistical Manual of Mental Disorders V,* 2013.

[4] Albert, U., et al., Suicide Risk in Obsessive-Compulsive Disorder and Exploration of Risk Factors: A Systematic Review. *Curr Neuropharmacol,* 2019. 17(8): p. 681-696.

[5] Wang, Y., et al., A screen of SLC1A1 for OCD-related alleles. *Am J Med Genet B Neuropsychiatr Genet,* 2010. 153B(2): p. 675-679.

[6] Dell'Osso, B., et al., Childhood, adolescent and adult age at onset and related clinical correlates in obsessive-compulsive disorder: a report from the International College of Obsessive-Compulsive Spectrum Disorders (ICOCS). *Int J Psychiatry Clin Pract,* 2016. 20(4): p. 210-7.

[7] Marazziti, D., et al., Increased inhibitory activity of protein kinase C on the serotonin transporter in OCD. *Neuropsychobiology,* 2000. 41(4): p. 171-7.

[8] Harvey, B.H., et al., Defining the neuromolecular action of myo-inositol: application to obsessive-compulsive disorder. *Prog Neuropsychopharmacol Biol Psychiatry,* 2002. 26(1): p. 21-32.

[9] Torres, A.R., et al., Obsessive-compulsive disorder: prevalence, comorbidity, impact, and help-seeking in the British National Psychiatric Morbidity Survey of 2000. *Am J Psychiatry,* 2006. 163(11): p. 1978-85.

[10] Pallanti, S. and G. Grassi, Pharmacologic treatment of obsessive-compulsive disorder comorbidity. *Expert Opin Pharmacother,* 2014. 15(17): p. 2543-52.

[11] Angst, J., et al., Obsessive-compulsive severity spectrum in the community: prevalence, comorbidity, and course. *Eur Arch Psychiatry Clin Neurosci,* 2004. 254(3): p. 156-64.

[12] Brakoulias, V., et al., Comorbidity, age of onset and suicidality in obsessive-compulsive disorder (OCD): An international collaboration. *Compr Psychiatry,* 2017. 76: p. 79-86.

[13] Ruscio, A.M., et al., The epidemiology of obsessive-compulsive disorder in the National Comorbidity Survey Replication. *Mol Psychiatry,* 2010. 15(1): p. 53-63.

[14] Schrag, A., et al., Streptococcal infection, Tourette syndrome, and OCD: is there a connection? *Neurology,* 2009. 73(16): p. 1256-63.

[15] Angst, J., et al., Suicide in 406 mood-disorder patients with and without long-term medication: a 40 to 44 years' follow-up. *Arch Suicide Res,* 2005. 9(3): p. 279-300.

[16] Nestadt, G., et al., Obsessive-compulsive disorder: subclassification based on co-morbidity. *Psychol Med,* 2009. 39(9): p. 1491-501.

[17] Eichstedt, J.A. and S.L. Arnold, Childhood-onset obsessive-compulsive disorder: a tic-related subtype of OCD? *Clin Psychol Rev,* 2001. 21(1): p. 137-57.

[18] Berrios, G.E., Our knowledge of anancasm (psychic compulsive states). *Hist Psychiatry,* 2003. 14(53 Pt 1): p. 113-28.

[19] Goodman, W.K., et al., Obsessive-compulsive disorder. *Psychiatr Clin North Am,* 2014. 37(3): p. 257-67.

[20] Mataix-Cols, D., M.C. Rosario-Campos, and J.F. Leckman, A multidimensional model of obsessive-compulsive disorder. *Am J Psychiatry,* 2005. 162(2): p. 228-38.

[21] Prado, H.S., et al., Sensory phenomena in obsessive-compulsive disorder and tic disorders: a review of the literature. *CNS Spectr,* 2008. 13(5): p. 425-32.

[22] Pallanti, S., et al., Obsessive-compulsive disorder comorbidity: clinical assessment and therapeutic implications. *Front Psychiatry,* 2011. 2: p. 70.

[23] Stein, D.J., et al., Meta-structure issues for the DSM-5: how do anxiety disorders, obsessive-compulsive and related disorders, post-traumatic disorders, and dissociative disorders fit together? *Curr Psychiatry Rep,* 2011. 13(4): p. 248-50.

[24] Van Ameringen, M., B. Patterson, and W. Simpson, DSM-5 obsessive-compulsive and related disorders: clinical implications of new criteria. *Depress Anxiety,* 2014. 31(6): p. 487-93.

[25] Leckman, J.F., et al., Obsessive-compulsive disorder: a review of the diagnostic criteria and possible subtypes and dimensional specifiers for DSM-V. *Depress Anxiety,* 2010. 27(6): p. 507-27.

[26] Mataix-Cols, D., A. Pertusa, and J.F. Leckman, Issues for DSM-V: how should obsessive-compulsive and related disorders be classified? *Am J Psychiatry,* 2007. 164(9): p. 1313-4.

[27] Nestadt, G., et al., The identification of OCD-related subgroups based on comorbidity. *Biol Psychiatry,* 2003. 53(10): p. 914-20.

[28] Lochner, C., et al., Cluster analysis of obsessive-compulsive spectrum disorders in patients with obsessive-compulsive disorder: clinical and genetic correlates. *Compr Psychiatry,* 2005. 46(1): p. 14-9.

[29] Association, A.P., *diagnostic and Statistical Manual of Mental Disorders* Fifth Edition American Psychiatric Press. 2013.

[30] Goodman, W.K., et al., The Yale-Brown Obsessive Compulsive Scale. I. Development, use, and reliability. *Arch Gen Psychiatry,* 1989. 46(11): p. 1006-11.

[31] Foa, E.B., et al., The Obsessive-Compulsive Inventory: development and validation of a short version. *Psychol Assess,* 2002. 14(4): p. 485-96.

[32] Prichep, L.S., et al., Quantitative electroencephalographic subtyping of obsessive-compulsive disorder. *Psychiatry Res,* 1993. 50(1): p. 25-32.

[33] Mas, F., et al., QEEG-LORETA Statistical Images of Obsessive Compulsive Disorder Heterogeneity. *NeuroImage,* 1998. 7(4, Part 2): p. S922.

[34] Bolwig, T.G., et al., Toward a better understanding of the pathophysiology of OCD SSRI responders: QEEG source localization. *Acta Psychiatr Scand,* 2007. 115(3): p. 237-42.

[35] Richter, P.M.A. and R.T. Ramos, Obsessive-Compulsive Disorder. Continuum (Minneap Minn), 2018. 24(3, *Behavioral Neurology and Psychiatry*): p. 828-844.

[36] Magalhaes, P.V., N.S. Kapczinski, and F. Kapczinski, Correlates and impact of obsessive-compulsive comorbidity in bipolar disorder. *Compr Psychiatry,* 2010. 51(4): p. 353-6.

[37] Kruger, S., et al., Comorbidity of obsessive compulsive disorder in bipolar disorder. *J Affect Disord,* 1995. 34(2): p. 117-20.

[38] McElroy, S.L., et al., Axis I psychiatric comorbidity and its relationship to historical illness variables in 288 patients with bipolar disorder. *Am J Psychiatry,* 2001. 158(3): p. 420-6.

[39] El-Mallakh, R.S. and M. Hollifield, Comorbid anxiety in bipolar disorder alters treatment and prognosis. *Psychiatr Q,* 2008. 79(2): p. 139-50.

[40] Perugi, G., et al., The clinical impact of bipolar and unipolar affective comorbidity on obsessive-compulsive disorder. *J Affect Disord,* 1997. 46(1): p. 15-23.

[41] Tukel, R., et al., Comorbid conditions in obsessive-compulsive disorder. *Compr Psychiatry,* 2002. 43(3): p. 204-9.

[42] D'Ambrosio, V., et al., Obsessive-compulsive disorder and cyclothymic temperament: an exploration of clinical features. *J Affect Disord,* 2010. 127(1-3): p. 295-9.

[43] Kruger, S., P. Braunig, and R.G. Cooke, Comorbidity of obsessive-compulsive disorder in recovered inpatients with bipolar disorder. *Bipolar Disord,* 2000. 2(1): p. 71-4.

[44] Hantouche, E.G., et al., Cyclothymic OCD: a distinct form? *J Affect Disord,* 2003. 75(1): p. 1-10.

[45] Hantouche, E.G., J. Angst, and H.S. Akiskal, Factor structure of hypomania: interrelationships with cyclothymia and the soft bipolar spectrum. *J Affect Disord,* 2003. 73(1-2): p. 39-47.

[46] Freeman, M.P., S.A. Freeman, and S.L. McElroy, The comorbidity of bipolar and anxiety disorders: prevalence, psychobiology, and treatment issues. *J Affect Disord,* 2002. 68(1): p. 1-23.

[47] Karno, M., et al., The epidemiology of obsessive-compulsive disorder in five US communities. *Arch Gen Psychiatry,* 1988. 45(12): p. 1094-9.

[48] Hwang, M.Y., et al., Treatment of schizophrenia with obsessive-compulsive features with serotonin reuptake inhibitors. *Am J Psychiatry,* 1993. 150(7): p. 1127.

[49] Lysaker, P.H. and K.A. Whitney, Obsessive-compulsive symptoms in schizophrenia: prevalence, correlates and treatment. *Expert Rev Neurother,* 2009. 9(1): p. 99-107.

[50] Saxena, S., et al., Neuroimaging and frontal-subcortical circuitry in obsessive-compulsive disorder. *Br J Psychiatry Suppl,* 1998(35): p. 26-37.

[51] Bloch, M.H., et al., A systematic review: antipsychotic augmentation with treatment refractory obsessive-compulsive disorder. *Mol Psychiatry,* 2006. 11(7): p. 622-32.

[52] Leckman, J.F., et al., Tic-related vs. non-tic-related obsessive compulsive disorder. *Anxiety,* 1994. 1(5): p. 208-15.

[53] Miguel, E.C., et al., Phenomenological differences appearing with repetitive behaviours in obsessive-compulsive disorder and Gilles de la Tourette's syndrome. *Br J Psychiatry,* 1997. 170: p. 140-5.

[54] di Michele, F., Utility of systematic studies of the immune function in obsessive-compulsive disorder patients. *Aust N Z J Psychiatry,* 2007. 41(5): p. 460-1.

[55] Alsheikh, A.M. and M.M. Alsheikh, Obsessive-Compulsive Disorder With Rheumatological and Inflammatory Diseases: A Systematic Review. *Cureus,* 2021. 13(5): p. e14791.

[56] Wang, L.Y., et al., Systemic autoimmune diseases are associated with an increased risk of obsessive-compulsive disorder: a nationwide population-based cohort study. *Soc Psychiatry Psychiatr Epidemiol,* 2019. 54(4): p. 507-516.

[57] Cosco, T.D., et al., Immune Aberrations in Obsessive-Compulsive Disorder: a Systematic Review and Meta-analysis. *Mol Neurobiol,* 2019. 56(7): p. 4751-4759.

[58] Jelinek, L., et al., Obsessive-compulsive disorder during COVID-19: Turning a problem into an opportunity? *J Anxiety Disord,* 2021. 77: p. 102329.

[59] Fineberg, N.A., et al., How to manage obsessive-compulsive disorder (OCD) under COVID-19: A clinician's guide from the International College of Obsessive Compulsive Spectrum Disorders (ICOCS) and the Obsessive-Compulsive and Related Disorders Research Network (OCRN) of the European College of Neuropsychopharmacology. *Compr Psychiatry,* 2020. 100: p. 152174.

[60] Lanciego, J.L. and A. Vazquez, The basal ganglia and thalamus of the long-tailed macaque in stereotaxic coordinates. A template atlas based on coronal, sagittal and horizontal brain sections. *Brain Struct Funct,* 2012. 217(2): p. 613-66.

[61] Nambu, A., Globus pallidus internal segment. *Prog Brain Res,* 2007. 160: p. 135-50.

[62] Benzina, N., et al., Cognitive Dysfunction in Obsessive-Compulsive Disorder. *Curr Psychiatry Rep,* 2016. 18(9): p. 80.

[63] O'Callaghan, C. and M. Hornberger, Towards a neurocomputational account of social dysfunction in neurodegenerative disease. *Brain,* 2017. 140(3): p. e14.

[64] Tian, L., et al., Abnormal functional connectivity of brain network hubs associated with symptom severity in treatment-naive patients with obsessive-compulsive disorder: A resting-state functional MRI study. *Prog Neuropsychopharmacol Biol Psychiatry,* 2016. 66: p. 104-111.

[65] van den Heuvel, M.P. and O. Sporns, Rich-club organization of the human connectome. *J Neurosci,* 2011. 31(44): p. 15775-86.

[66] Yun, J.Y., et al., Brain structural covariance networks in obsessive-compulsive disorder: a graph analysis from the ENIGMA Consortium. *Brain,* 2020. 143(2): p. 684-700.

[67] Purcell, R., et al., Neuropsychological deficits in obsessive-compulsive disorder: a comparison with unipolar depression, panic disorder, and normal controls. *Arch Gen Psychiatry,* 1998. 55(5): p. 415-23.

[68] Cummings, J.L. and K. Cunningham, Obsessive-compulsive disorder in Huntington's disease. *Biol Psychiatry,* 1992. 31(3): p. 263-70.

[69] Piallat, B., et al., Subthalamic neuronal firing in obsessive-compulsive disorder and Parkinson disease. *Ann Neurol,* 2011. 69(5): p. 793-802.

[70] Park, Y.S., et al., Anatomic Review of the Ventral Capsule/Ventral Striatum and the Nucleus Accumbens to Guide Target Selection for Deep Brain Stimulation for Obsessive-Compulsive Disorder. *World Neurosurg,* 2019. 126: p. 1-10.

[71] Hoppenbrouwers, S.S., et al., The role of the cerebellum in the pathophysiology and treatment of neuropsychiatric disorders: a review. *Brain Res Rev,* 2008. 59(1): p. 185-200.

[72] Miquel, M., et al., A Working Hypothesis for the Role of the Cerebellum in Impulsivity and Compulsivity. *Front Behav Neurosci,* 2019. 13: p. 99.

[73] Bandelow, B., et al., Biological markers for anxiety disorders, OCD and PTSD: A consensus statement. Part II: Neurochemistry, neurophysiology and neurocognition. *World J Biol Psychiatry,* 2017. 18(3): p. 162-214.

[74] Delgado, P.L. and F.A. Moreno, Hallucinogens, serotonin and obsessive-compulsive disorder. *J Psychoactive Drugs,* 1998. 30(4): p. 359-66.

[75] Bergqvist, P.B., J. Dong, and P. Blier, Effect of atypical antipsychotic drugs on 5-HT2 receptors in the rat orbito-frontal cortex: an in vivo electrophysiological study. *Psychopharmacology (Berl),* 1999. 143(1): p. 89-96.

[76] el Mansari, M., C. Bouchard, and P. Blier, Alteration of serotonin release in the guinea pig orbito-frontal cortex by selective serotonin reuptake inhibitors. Relevance to treatment of obsessive-

compulsive disorder. *Neuropsychopharmacology,* 1995. 13(2): p. 117-27.

[77] Taylor, S., Molecular genetics of obsessive-compulsive disorder: a comprehensive meta-analysis of genetic association studies. *Mol Psychiatry,* 2013. 18(7): p. 799-805.

[78] Taylor, S., Disorder-specific genetic factors in obsessive-compulsive disorder: A comprehensive meta-analysis. *Am J Med Genet B Neuropsychiatr Genet,* 2016. 171B(3): p. 325-32.

[79] Nikolaus, S., et al., Cortical GABA, striatal dopamine and midbrain serotonin as the key players in compulsive and anxiety disorders--results from in vivo imaging studies. *Rev Neurosci,* 2010. 21(2): p. 119-39.

[80] Olver, J.S., et al., Dopamine D(1) receptor binding in the anterior cingulate cortex of patients with obsessive-compulsive disorder. *Psychiatry Res,* 2010. 183(1): p. 85-8.

[81] Pittenger, C., M.H. Bloch, and K. Williams, Glutamate abnormalities in obsessive compulsive disorder: neurobiology, pathophysiology, and treatment. *Pharmacol Ther,* 2011. 132(3): p. 314-32.

[82] Bhattacharyya, S., et al., Anti-brain autoantibodies and altered excitatory neurotransmitters in obsessive-compulsive disorder. *Neuropsychopharmacology,* 2009. 34(12): p. 2489-96.

[83] Chakrabarty, K., et al., Glutamatergic dysfunction in OCD. *Neuropsychopharmacology,* 2005. 30(9): p. 1735-40.

[84] Arnold, P.D., et al., Glutamate transporter gene SLC1A1 associated with obsessive-compulsive disorder. *Arch Gen Psychiatry,* 2006. 63(7): p. 769-76.

[85] Mattheisen, M., et al., Genome-wide association study in obsessive-compulsive disorder: results from the OCGAS. *Mol Psychiatry,* 2015. 20(3): p. 337-44.

[86] Varma, A.R., et al., HMPAO SPECT in non-epileptic seizures: preliminary results. *Acta Neurol Scand,* 1996. 94(2): p. 88-92.

[87] Stewart, S.E., et al., Meta-analysis of association between obsessive-compulsive disorder and the 3' region of neuronal

glutamate transporter gene SLC1A1. *Am J Med Genet B Neuropsychiatr Genet,* 2013. 162B(4): p. 367-79.
[88] Mundo, E., et al., Is the 5-HT(1Dbeta) receptor gene implicated in the pathogenesis of obsessive-compulsive disorder? *Am J Psychiatry,* 2000. 157(7): p. 1160-1.
[89] Nicolini, H., et al., [Dopamine D2 and D4 receptor genes distinguish the clinical presence of tics in obsessive-compulsive disorder]. *Gac Med Mex,* 1998. 134(5): p. 521-7.
[90] International Obsessive Compulsive Disorder Foundation Genetics, C. and O.C.D.C.G.A. Studies, Revealing the complex genetic architecture of obsessive-compulsive disorder using meta-analysis. *Mol Psychiatry,* 2018. 23(5): p. 1181-1188.
[91] NICE, National Institute for Health and Care Excellence. 2013.
[92] Deacon, B.J. and J.S. Abramowitz, Cognitive and behavioral treatments for anxiety disorders: A review of meta-analytic findings. *Journal of clinical psychology,* 2004. 60(4): p. 429-441.
[93] Association, A.P., et al., *Practice guideline for the treatment of patients with obsessive-compulsive disorder.* 2007.
[94] Pittenger, C. and M.H. Bloch, Pharmacological treatment of obsessive-compulsive disorder. *Psychiatric Clinics,* 2014. 37(3): p. 375-391.
[95] Ackerman, D.L. and S. Greenland, Multivariate meta-analysis of controlled drug studies for obsessive-compulsive disorder. *Journal of clinical psychopharmacology,* 2002. 22(3): p. 309-317.
[96] Simpson, H.B., et al., Response versus remission in obsessive-compulsive disorder. *The Journal of clinical psychiatry,* 2006. 67(2): p. 0-0.
[97] Fineberg, N.A., et al., Sustained response versus relapse: the pharmacotherapeutic goal for obsessive–compulsive disorder. *International clinical psychopharmacology,* 2007. 22(6): p. 313-322.
[98] Fineberg, N.A., et al., Escitalopram prevents relapse of obsessive-compulsive disorder. *European neuropsychopharmacology,* 2007. 17(6-7): p. 430-439.

[99] Dold, M., et al., Antipsychotic augmentation of serotonin reuptake inhibitors in treatment-resistant obsessive-compulsive disorder: a meta-analysis of double-blind, randomized, placebo-controlled trials. *International Journal of Neuropsychopharmacology,* 2013. 16(3): p. 557-574.

[100] Donovan, M.R., et al., Comparative efficacy of antidepressants in preventing relapse in anxiety disorders—a meta-analysis. *Journal of affective disorders,* 2010. 123(1-3): p. 9-16.

[101] Carmi, L., et al., Efficacy and safety of deep transcranial magnetic stimulation for obsessive-compulsive disorder: a prospective multicenter randomized double-blind placebo-controlled trial. *American Journal of Psychiatry,* 2019. 176(11): p. 931-938.

[102] Soomro, G.M., et al., Selective serotonin re-uptake inhibitors (SSRIs) versus placebo for obsessive compulsive disorder (OCD). *Cochrane database of systematic reviews,* 2008(1).

[103] McDougle, C.J., et al., Limited therapeutic effect of addition of buspirone in fluvoxamine-refractory obsessive-compulsive disorder. *The American journal of psychiatry,* 1993.

[104] McDOUGLE, C.J., et al., A controlled trial of lithium augmentation in fluvoxamine-refractory obsessive-compulsive disorder: lack of efficacy. *Journal of Clinical Psychopharmacology,* 1991.

[105] Stern, E.R., et al., High-dose ondansetron reduces activation of interoceptive and sensorimotor brain regions. *Neuropsychopharmacology,* 2019. 44(2): p. 390-398.

[106] Saxena, S., et al., Localized orbitofrontal and subcortical metabolic changes and predictors of response to paroxetine treatment in obsessive-compulsive disorder. *Neuropsychopharmacology,* 1999. 21(6): p. 683-693.

[107] Landeros-Weisenberger, A., et al., Dimensional predictors of response to SRI pharmacotherapy in obsessive–compulsive disorder. *Journal of affective disorders,* 2010. 121(1-2): p. 175-179.

[108] Saxena, S., et al., Differential brain metabolic predictors of response to paroxetine in obsessive-compulsive disorder versus major depression. *American Journal of Psychiatry,* 2003. 160(3): p. 522-532.

[109] Hollander, E., et al., Acute and long-term treatment and prevention of relapse of obsessive-compulsive disorder with paroxetine. *The Journal of clinical psychiatry,* 2003. 64(9): p. 0-0.

[110] Stein, M.B., et al., Fluvoxamine treatment of social phobia (social anxiety disorder): a double-blind, placebo-controlled study. *American Journal of Psychiatry,* 1999. 156(5): p. 756-760.

[111] Szegedi, A., et al., Combination treatment with clomipramine and fluvoxamine: drug monitoring, safety, and tolerability data. *The Journal of clinical psychiatry,* 1996. 57(6): p. 257-264.

[112] Montgomery, S., et al., Citalopram 20 mg, 40 mg and 60 mg are all effective and well tolerated compared with placebo in obsessive-compulsive disorder. *International clinical psychopharmacology,* 2001. 16(2): p. 75-86.

[113] *FDA Drug Safety Communication: Revised recommendations for Celexa (citalopram hydrobromide) related to a potential risk of abnormal heart rhythms with high doses.* 2017.

[114] Bloch, M.H., et al., Meta-analysis of the dose-response relationship of SSRI in obsessive-compulsive disorder. *Molecular psychiatry,* 2010. 15(8): p. 850-855.

[115] Phillips, K.A. and S.A. Rasmussen, Change in psychosocial functioning and quality of life of patients with body dysmorphic disorder treated with fluoxetine: a placebo-controlled study. *Psychosomatics,* 2004. 45(5): p. 438-444.

[116] Liebowitz, M.R., et al., Efficacy of sertraline in severe generalized social anxiety disorder: results of a double-blind, placebo-controlled study. *The Journal of clinical psychiatry,* 2003. 64(7): p. 0-0.

[117] Ninan, P.T., et al., High-dose sertraline strategy for nonresponders to acute treatment for obsessive-compulsive disorder: a multicenter

double-blind trial. *The Journal of clinical psychiatry,* 2006. 67(1): p. 0-0.

[118] Greist, J.H., et al., Clomipramine and obsessive compulsive disorder: a placebo-controlled double-blind study of 32 patients. *The Journal of clinical psychiatry,* 1990.

[119] FALLON, B.A. and S.J. MATHEW, Biological therapies for obsessive-compulsive disorder. *Journal of Psychiatric Practice®,* 2000. 6(3): p. 113-128.

[120] Hollander, E., et al., Venlafaxine in treatment-resistant obsessive-compulsive disorder. *Journal of Clinical Psychiatry,* 2003. 64(5): p. 546-550.

[121] Phelps, N.J. and M.E. Cates, The Role of Venlafaxine in the Treatment of Obsessive—Compulsive Disorder. *Annals of Pharmacotherapy,* 2005. 39(1): p. 136-140.

[122] Balachander, S., et al., Effectiveness of Venlafaxine in Selective Serotonin Reuptake Inhibitor–Resistant Obsessive-Compulsive Disorder: Experience From a Specialty Clinic in India. *Journal of clinical psychopharmacology,* 2019. 39(1): p. 82-85.

[123] Dell'Osso, B., et al., Switching from serotonin reuptake inhibitors to duloxetine in patients with resistant obsessive compulsive disorder: a case series. *Journal of Psychopharmacology,* 2008. 22(2): p. 210-213.

[124] Marazziti, D., et al., Effectiveness of long-term augmentation with citalopram to clomipramine in treatment-resistant OCD patients. *CNS spectrums,* 2008. 13(11): p. 971-976.

[125] Ravizza, L., et al., Drug treatment of obsessive-compulsive disorder (OCD): long-term trial with clomipramine and selective serotonin reuptake inhibitors (SSRIs). *Psychopharmacology bulletin,* 1996.

[126] Ravindran, L., S. Jung, and A. Ravindran, Intravenous anti-obsessive agents: a review. *Journal of Psychopharmacology,* 2010. 24(3): p. 287-296.

[127] Albert, U., et al., A systematic review of evidence-based treatment strategies for obsessive-compulsive disorder resistant to first-line

pharmacotherapy. *Current medicinal chemistry,* 2018. 25(41): p. 5647-5661.

[128] Berlin, H.A., et al., Double-blind, placebo-controlled trial of topiramate augmentation in treatment-resistant obsessive-compulsive disorder. *The Journal of clinical psychiatry,* 2010. 71(5): p. 0-0.

[129] Uzun, Ö., Lamotrigine as an augmentation agent in treatment-resistant obsessive-compulsive disorder: a case report. *Journal of psychopharmacology,* 2010. 24(3): p. 425-427.

[130] Arrojo-Romero, M., M. Tajes Alonso, and J. de Leon, Lamotrigine augmentation of serotonin reuptake inhibitors in severe and long-term treatment-resistant obsessive-compulsive disorder. *Case reports in psychiatry,* 2013. 2013.

[131] Mowla, A., et al., Topiramate augmentation in resistant OCD: a double-blind placebo-controlled clinical trial. *CNS spectrums,* 2010. 15(11): p. 613-617.

[132] Önder, E., Ü. Tural, and M. Gökbakan, Does gabapentin lead to early symptom improvement in obsessive-compulsive disorder? European archives of psychiatry and clinical neuroscience, 2008. 258(6): p. 319-323.

[133] Marinova, Z., D.-M. Chuang, and N. Fineberg, Glutamate-modulating drugs as a potential therapeutic strategy in obsessive-compulsive disorder. *Current Neuropharmacology,* 2017. 15(7): p. 977-995.

[134] Ghaleiha, A., et al., Memantine add-on in moderate to severe obsessive-compulsive disorder: randomized double-blind placebo-controlled study. *Journal of psychiatric research,* 2013. 47(2): p. 175-180.

[135] Rodriguez, C.I., et al., Randomized controlled crossover trial of ketamine in obsessive-compulsive disorder: proof-of-concept. *Neuropsychopharmacology,* 2013. 38(12): p. 2475-2483.

[136] Pittenger, C., et al., Riluzole augmentation in treatment-refractory obsessive-compulsive disorder: a pilot randomized placebo-

controlled trial. *The Journal of clinical psychiatry,* 2015. 76(8): p. 0-0.

[137] Coric, V., et al., Riluzole augmentation in treatment-resistant obsessive–compulsive disorder: an open-label trial. *Biological psychiatry,* 2005. 58(5): p. 424-428.

[138] Paydary, K., et al., N-acetylcysteine augmentation therapy for moderate-to-severe obsessive–compulsive disorder: Randomized, double-blind, placebo-controlled trial. *Journal of clinical pharmacy and therapeutics,* 2016. 41(2): p. 214-219.

[139] di Michele, F., In Nova ed. *Therapeutic use of N-Acetylcisteine for obsessive-compulsive disorder: a new avenue,* 2020.

[140] Serata, D., et al., Are 5-HT3 antagonists effective in obsessive–compulsive disorder? A systematic review of literature. *Human Psychopharmacology: Clinical and Experimental,* 2015. 30(2): p. 70-84.

[141] Liddell, M.B., et al., Buprenorphine augmentation in the treatment of refractory obsessive–compulsive disorder. *Therapeutic Advances in Psychopharmacology,* 2013. 3(1): p. 15-19.

[142] Andersson, E., et al., D-cycloserine vs placebo as adjunct to cognitive behavioral therapy for obsessive-compulsive disorder and interaction with antidepressants: a randomized clinical trial. *JAMA psychiatry,* 2015. 72(7): p. 659-667.

[143] Blessing, E.M., et al., Cannabidiol as a potential treatment for anxiety disorders. *Neurotherapeutics,* 2015. 12(4): p. 825-836.

[144] Öst, L.-G., et al., Cognitive behavioral and pharmacological treatments of OCD in children: A systematic review and meta-analysis. *Journal of Anxiety Disorders,* 2016. 43: p. 58-69.

[145] Invernizzi, G. and C. Bressi, *Manuale di psichiatria e psicologia clinica.* 2012: Mc Graw Hill. [*Manual of Psychiatry and Clinical Psychology.*]

[146] Rogers, M.A., et al., Internet-delivered health interventions that work: systematic review of meta-analyses and evaluation of website availability. *Journal of medical Internet research,* 2017. 19(3): p. e7111.

[147] Krzyszkowiak, W., M. Kuleta-Krzyszkowiak, and E. Krzanowska, Treatment of obsessive-compulsive disorders (OCD) and obsessive-compulsive-related disorders (OCRD). *Psychiatria polska,* 2019. 53(4): p. 825-843.

[148] Berlim, M.T., N.H. Neufeld, and F. Van den Eynde, Repetitive transcranial magnetic stimulation (rTMS) for obsessive-compulsive disorder (OCD): An exploratory meta-analysis of randomized and sham-controlled trials. *Journal of psychiatric research,* 2013. 47(8): p. 999-1006.

[149] Trevizol, A.P., et al., Transcranial magnetic stimulation for obsessive-compulsive disorder: an updated systematic review and meta-analysis. *The journal of ECT,* 2016. 32(4): p. 262-266.

[150] Lusicic, A., et al., Transcranial magnetic stimulation in the treatment of obsessive–compulsive disorder: current perspectives. *Neuropsychiatric disease and treatment,* 2018. 14: p. 1721.

[151] Haber, S.N., The primate basal ganglia: parallel and integrative networks. *Journal of chemical neuroanatomy,* 2003. 26(4): p. 317-330.

[152] Maia, T.V., R.E. Cooney, and B.S. Peterson, The neural bases of obsessive–compulsive disorder in children and adults. *Development and psychopathology,* 2008. 20(4): p. 1251-1283.

[153] Van Veen, V. and C.S. Carter, The anterior cingulate as a conflict monitor: fMRI and ERP studies. *Physiology & behavior,* 2002. 77(4-5): p. 477-482.

[154] Sheth, S.A., et al., Limbic system surgery for treatment-refractory obsessive-compulsive disorder: a prospective long-term follow-up of 64 patients. *Journal of neurosurgery,* 2013. 118(3): p. 491-497.

[155] Miguel, E.C., et al., Evolution of gamma knife capsulotomy for intractable obsessive-compulsive disorder. *Molecular psychiatry,* 2019. 24(2): p. 218-240.

[156] Goodman, W.K. and R.L. Alterman, Deep brain stimulation for intractable psychiatric disorders. *Annual review of medicine,* 2012. 63: p. 511-524.

BIOGRAPHICAL SKETCHES

Riccardo Santini

Affiliation:

- Chair of Psychiatry, Department of Systems Medicine, University of Rome Tor Vergata, Rome, Italy
- Psychiatry and Clinical Psychology Unit, Fondazione Policlinico Tor Vergata, Rome, Italy

Education:

- Graduated from "Università degli Studi di Roma La Sapienza" Medical School;
- Psichiatry Residency Program at University of "Tor Vergata", Rome

Research and Professional Experience: Erasmus Programme at Universitatea de Medicină şi farmacie "Grigore T. Popa", Iaşi (Romania) (2017-2018)

Publications from the Last 3 Years:

1. Fiori Nastro F., Mariano A., Pelle M., Santini R., di Michele F., Bianchi F., Niolu C., Siracusano A.; *Comparison of psychiatric emergency service admission rates in an Italian Covid-19 Hospital during lockdown and last year*; (European Congress EPA 2020).

Antonella Mariano

Affiliation:

- Chair of Psychiatry, Department of Systems Medicine, University of Rome Tor Vergata, Rome, Italy.
- Psychiatry and Clinical Psychology Unit, Fondazione Policlinico Tor Vergata, Rome, Italy.

Education:

- Graduated from "Università degli Studi di Roma La Sapienza" Medical School;
- Psichiatry Residency Program at University of "Tor Vergata", Rome

Research and Professional Experience:

- Erasmus Programme at Rheinische Friedrich-Wilhelms-Universität, Bonn (Germany) (2016-2017)
- Traineeship in Infantile Epilepsy Evangelisches Krankenhaus Königin Elisabeth Herzberge, Berlin (Germany)

Publications from the Last 3 Years:

1. Fiori Nastro F., Mariano A., Pelle M., Santini R., di Michele F., Bianchi F., Niolu C., Siracusano A.; *Comparison of psychiatric emergency service admission rates in an Italian Covid-19 Hospital during lockdown and last year*; (European Congress EPA 2020).

Federico Fiori Nastro

Affiliation:

- Chair of Psychiatry, Department of Systems Medicine, University of Rome Tor Vergata, Rome, Italy
- Psychiatry and Clinical Psychology Unit, Fondazione Policlinico Tor Vergata, Rome, Italy

Education:

- Graduated from "Università degli Studi di Roma La Sapienza" Medical School;
- Psichiatry Residency Program at University of "Tor Vergata", Rome

Research and Professional Experience:

- Medical Elective at Saint Mary Hospital, Imperial College London (UK), Child and Adolescent Mental Health Service

Publications from the Last 3 Years:

1. Fiori Nastro F., Mariano A., Pelle M., Santini R., di Michele F., Bianchi F., Niolu C., Siracusano A.; *Comparison of psychiatric emergency service admission rates in an Italian Covid-19 Hospital during lockdown and last year*; (European Congress EPA 2020);
2. Fiori Nastro F., Croce D., Schmidt S.J., Michel C. Basili R., Schultze-Lutter F.; *Inside Out Project: using Big Data and Machine Learning for Prevention in Psychiatry*; (European Congress EPA 2020).
3. Fiori Nastro F., Pelle M., di Michele F., Talamo A., Niolu C., Siracusano A.; *A Cross-Sectional Study on outcomes of*

individuals with first Hospitalization and psychosis spectrum disorder diagnosis, Schizophrenia Research (SIRS Congress Florence 4-8 April 2020).
4. Pelle M., Fiori Nastro F., di Michele F., Talamo A., Siracusano A., Niolu C., *L'aggressività nel paziente psichiatrico in acuzie: prevalenza e correlazioni con variabili cliniche e sociodemografiche,* (SIP Giovani 2020). [*Aggression in acute psychiatric patients: prevalence and correlations with clinical and socio-demographic variables*]
5. Basili R., Bellomaria V., Bugge N.J., Croce D., De Michele F., Fiori Nastro F., Fiori Nastro P., Michel C., Schmidt S.J., Schultze-Lutter F.; *Monitoring Adolescents' Distress using Social Web data as a Source: the InsideOut Project*, dblp computer scienze bibliography 2017.
6. Fiori Nastro F., De Michele F., *Big data Machine Learning e Intelligenza Artificiale: nuove prospettive per la prevenzione in psichiatria*. L'esperienza del Progetto InsideOut, Il Sogno della Farfalla, 4, 2018.

Martina Pelle

Affiliation:

- Chair of Psychiatry, Department of Systems Medicine, University of Rome Tor Vergata, Rome, Italy
- Psychiatry and Clinical Psychology Unit, Fondazione Policlinico Tor Vergata, Rome, Italy

Education:

- Graduated from "Università degli Studi di Roma La Sapienza" Medical School;

- Psichiatry Residency Program at University of "Tor Vergata", Rome

Publications from the Last 3 Years:

1. Fiori Nastro F., Mariano A., Pelle M., Santini R., di Michele F., Bianchi F., Niolu C., Siracusano A.; *Comparison of psychiatric emergency service admission rates in an Italian Covid-19 Hospital during lockdown and last year*; (European Congress EPA 2020).
2. Fiori Natsro F., Pelle M., di Michele F., Talamo A., Niolu C., Siracusano A.; *A Cross-Sectional Study on outcomes of individuals with first Hospitalization and psychosis spectrum disorder diagnosis,* Schizophrenia Research (SIRS Congress Florence 4-8 April 2020).
3. Pelle M., Fiori Nastro F., di Michele F., Talamo A., Siracusano A., Niolu C., *L'aggressività nel paziente psichiatrico in acuzie: prevalenza e correlazioni con variabili cliniche e sociodemografiche,* SIP Giovani 2020. [*Aggression in acute psychiatric patients: prevalence and correlations with clinical and socio-demographic variables*]
4. Bianciardi E., Imperatori C., Innamorati M., Fabbricatori M., Monacelli M.A., Pelle M., Siracusano A., Niolu C., Gentileschi P.; *Measuring Knowledge, Attitudes and Barriers to Medication Adherence in Potential Bariatric Surgery Patients*; Obesity Surgery 2021.

Flavia di Michele

Affiliation: Psychiatry and Clinical Psychology Unit, Fondazione Policlinico Tor Vergata, Rome, Italy

Education:

- Graduated from "Tor Vergata University of Rome" School of Medicine, 1995;
- Residency in Psychiatry at University of "Tor Vergata" of Rome, 1999;
- PhD program in Neuroscience at Tor Vergata University of Rome, 2006.

Professional and Research Experience:

- Jan 2017-Present: Psychiatrist at UOC Psychiatry and Psychology, Dept Systems Medicine, Policlinico Tor Vergata Foundation, Rome, Italy.
- Dec. 2013-Dec.2016: Psychiatrist at the Acute Psychiatric Unit of Ospedale di Sora (FR)
- May 2011-Dec.2013: Psychiatrist at the Acute Psychiatric Unit of Ospedale Grassi, Rome
- Sept.2010-Apr.2011: Psychiatrist at the Mental Health Dept of Tarquinia and Viterbo (VT)
- Sept.2006-Aug.2010: Psychiatrist at the Mental Health Dept of Ariano Irpino (AV)
- June 2004-Aug.2006: Psychiatrist at the Mental Health Dept of ASL Napoli 5 (NA)
- Jan 2000-May 2004: Psychiatrist at the Mental Health Dept of ASL Rome B-C-D-E and for the Italian Army Service.
- 1994-2007: Neuroscience Researcher at IRCCS Santa Lucia, Rome, Neuroendocrinol labs directed by Dr. E. Romeo, in collaboration with the team of Prof Rupprecht of the Max Planck Institute of Munich, Germany.

Teaching Activities:

- 2017-present: Tutor of resident students in psychiatry at the Acute Psychiatric Unit of PTV Foundation, for Tor Vergata University.
- 2014: Teacher in the master program organized by the ASL of Frosinone on Mood disorders, Anxiety and Obsessive-Compulsive Disorders.
- 2006-2010: Teacher in the course for Physiotherapists of Second University of Naples of Child and Adolescent neuropsychiatry.
- 2001: Teacher in the course of Psychogeriatry on neuropsychopharmacology organized by the IRCSS S. Lucia of Rome.
- Author of more than 62 scientific works (publications, chapters in books and conference papers).
- Peer Reviewer for the following Journals: "Journal of Clinical Psychiatry", "Journal of Psychiatry and Neuroscience", since 2006; "JNNP" since 2011; "Canadian Journal of Psychiatry" since 2015; "Psychoneuroendocrinology" since 2017; "Brasilian J Psychiatry" since 2021; "Primary Health Care Development" since 2021. Guest Editor for "Current Pharmaceutical Design", 2020-

Publications from the Last 3 Years:

1. di Michele F., A. Siracusano, A. Talamo, C. Niolu. N-Acetyl cysteine and Vitamin D supplementation in treatment resistant Obsessive-compulsive disorder patients: a general review. *Curr Pharm Des,* 24(17):1832-1838, 2018. doi: 10.2174/1381612824 666180417124919.
2. di Michele F. Vitamin D supplementation in Obsessive-compulsive disorder. *Psychiatry Res,* 270:1174, 2018. doi: 10.1016/j.psychres.2018.06.059.
3. di Michele F., A. Talamo, C. Niolu, A. Siracusano. Vitamin D and N-Acetyl cysteine supplementation in treatment resistant

Depression: a general review. *Curr Pharm Des,* 26(21):2442-2459, 2020. doi: 10.2174/1381612826666200406090051.
4. di Michele F. Why Vitamin D is important for wellbeing and mental health. Editorial. *Curr Pharm Des,* 26(21):2439-2441, 2020.
5. Brogna P., R. Colasuonno, F. di Michele, A. Paterniti, A. Talamo, Ribolsi M., C. Niolu, A. Siracusano. Diagnostic and therapeutic challenges in Neuroleptic Malignant Syndrome: a severe medical case. *Rivista di Psichiatria,* 55(4):236-239, 2020.
6. Niolu C., Talamo A., Caporusso E., di Michele F., Brogna N., D'Argenio A., Paterniti A., Facchi A., Infante V., Liberato D., Miri Lavasani D., Pomilio A., Tomassini L., Siracusano A. *Vitamin D Supplement Therapy among hospitalized patients with psychosis spectrum disorder: clinical and therapeutic correlates.* Abstr in EPA, Nice, March, Vol. 48 pp S726, 2018.
7. Niolu C., Talamo A., Lombardozzi G., Colasuonno R., Coviello M., Palazzetti C., di Michele F., Brogna P., D'Argenio A., Paterniti A., Facchi A., Infante V., Urso S., Lisi G., Riconi A., Amodeo A., Marsella, Milano F., Siracusano A. *Violent behavior in acute psychiatric inpatients: Clinical characteristics, neuropsychological and therapeutic correlates.* Abstr in ECNP, Barcelona, Oct. 2018.
8. Amodeo A., Talamo A., Riconi A., Contini L., Coviello M., Adulti I., di Michele F., Brogna P., D'Argenio A., Paterniti A., Facchi A., Infante V., Tarantino G., Lisi N., Procinesi C., Siracusano A., Niolu C. *A framework based on the Research Domain Criteria (RDoC) comparing individuals with severe mental illness with and without history of child sexual abuse: Clinical Evaluation and Characteristics.* Abstr in EPA, Warsaw, April, 2019.
9. Talamo A., Fiorinastro F., Pelle M., Di Mario A., Medici C., Di Francia A., Sacchetto S., Felici R., Rinaldi F., di Michele F., Brogna P., D'Argenio A., Paterniti A., Infante V., Siracusano A., Niolu C. *Recent stressful life events and relation to an acute*

psychiatric episode among individuals with severe mental illness: sociodemographic and clinical characteristics. Abstr in EPA, Madrid 2020.
10. Fiorinastro F., Pelle M. di Michele F., Talamo A., Siracusano A., Niolu C. *A Cross-Sectional Study on outcomes of individuals with first hospitalization and psychosis spectrum disorder diagnosis.* Abstr in SIRS, Florence 2020 published on *Schizophrenia Bulletin* 46(Suppl_1):S275-S276. May 2020.
11. Pelle M., Fiorinastro F., di Michele F., Talamo A., Siracusano A., Niolu C. *L'aggressività nel paziente psichiatrico in acuzie: prevalenza e correlazione con variabili cliniche e sociodemografiche.* Abst in SIP giovani, Rome 2020. [*Aggression in acute psychiatric patients: prevalence and correlation with clinical and socio-demographic variables.*]
12. Fiori Nastro F., Mariano A., Pelle M., Santini R., di Michele F., Bianchi F., Niolu C., Siracusano A. *Comparison of psychiatric emergency service admission rates in an Italian Covid-19 Hospital during lockdown and last year;* European Congress EPA 2021.
13. di Michele F. Therapeutic use of N-Acetylcisteine for Obsessive Compulsive Disorder treatment: a new avenue. In *"Cysteine: Sources, Uses and Health Effects."* Pp. Eds. Nova 2021.
14. di Michele, F. Why use nutraceutical strategies for the Irritable Bowel Syndrome. *Curr Med Chem,* in press.
15. di Michele, F., A. Talamo, G. Di Lorenzo, C. Niolu, A. Siracusano. Psychiatric and neurological management of severe acute psychomotor agitation: A rare case of an adult presentation of Rasmussen Syndrome. *Riv Psichiatria,* in press.

In: Obsessive-Compulsive Disorder
Editor: Jeffrey L. Nelson

ISBN: 978-1-68507-310-7
© 2021 Nova Science Publishers, Inc.

Chapter 2

RELEVANT MECHANISMS IN TREATING OBSESSIVE-COMPULSIVE DISORDER: THE CASE FOR DOMAIN-SPECIFIC RELEVANCE WITH SCRUPULOSITY AND OTHER FORMS OF OBSESSIONS AND COMPULSIONS

Dakota Mauzay[*], *PhD*
University of Idaho Counseling and Testing Center,
Moscow, Idaho, USA

ABSTRACT

Contrary to popular representations of obsessive-compulsive disorder (OCD), OCD is a highly heterogeneous presentation. As such,

---

[*] Corresponding Author's E-mail: drmauzay@gmail.com.

there are a variety of clinical constructs and hypothesized mechanisms of action clinicians need to consider when working with OCD. This is of paramount importance as the body of knowledge within the treatment literature of OCD grows and continued differences between symptom subtypes of OCD are observed. Indeed, it is possible that varying presentations of OCD may have different mechanisms of action. Further, personal and cultural factors have been articulated as being relevant to the treatment of differing subtypes of OCD. Although there is a growing body of evidence indicating some treatments can be a highly effective means of treating OCD, it is important to note that even highly effective treatments often leave many still suffering from their obsessions and compulsions. Further, the possibility for homogeneous treatments of OCD to result in a "one size fits all" mentality necessitates continued attention being given to the aforementioned areas of OCD discussed. The present writing explores some of the nuisances present in working with individuals with OCD within the context of obsessive and compulsive content that may require additive elements to be considered in treatment. Particular attention is given to scrupulosity and factors relevant within the treatment of scrupulosity.

INTRODUCTION

Obsessive-compulsive disorder is characterized by either obsessions and/or compulsions generally and can often result in an individual having an expansive heterogenious, idiosyncratic clinical presentation (American Psychiatric Association, 2013; Lochner et al., 2008; Schalkwyk et al., 2016). Contrary to some representations of OCD, this diagnosis is a highly heterogeneous presentation that can be expressed in varying clinical subtypes which poses challenges for researchers and clinicians alike (Lochner et al., 2008). Religious and moral obsessions and compulsions, often referred to as scrupulosity, is one particular example of a unique subtype of OCD. Some authors discuss scrupulosity in the context of religiosity primarily (e.g., Abramowitz & Jacoby, 2014), but in the current writing it will be used to describe obsessions and compulsions that are religious or moral in nature, or that involve engaging in actions deemed immoral by the individual broadly defined (e.g., physical and sexual aggression). There are a variety of models addressing symptom manifestation and maintenance among individuals with OCD. Psychologically, two of the most well-known and studied models are the behavioral and cognitive models of OCD, with a variety of smaller models encompassed within these two existing to explain OCD symptom manifestation and treatment. Many of the behavioral models of OCD consist of examining the role of operant processes within the development of OCD symptoms. For instance, through the behavioral model, OCD symptoms are conceptualized as being maintained through the negative reinforcement that occurs when an individual engages in compulsions to reduce distress from an obsession at the expense of long-term symptom worsening (Cassin & Rector, 2011; Foa, 2010). This process has been argued to occur as a function of various behavioral or even cognitive processes (Cassin & Rector; Foa, 2010). Still, although the etiological mechanisms may vary, the proposed form of treatment is often exposure and response prevention (ERP; Cassin & Rector, 2011; Foa, 2010). Therefore, the behavioral model of treatment is one in which the individual is exposed to their obsessions while refraining from engaging in compulsive actions or other processes that will assist the individual in avoiding the distress associated with the exposure (Cassin & Rector, 2011; Foa, 2010). The way in which compulsions are utilized to provide temporary, short-term relief to the individual often takes one of two forms. Firstly, Cassin and Rector (2011) posit that compulsions are used to prevent an outcome associated with the individual's obsessions coming to fruition. Secondly, the authors argue that compulsions can serve in facilitating the individual feeling as though their compulsive behavioral or mental actions have been fully completed (Cassin & Rector, 2011). Although elements of both the behavioral and cognitive theories of OCD are often intertwined heavily to the extent that it can be hard to disentangle them, the more cognitive-based interpretation of OCD symptom development puts greater emphasis on the role of cognitive misinterpretations and mechanisms that underlie symptoms of OCD (Rachman, 1997). Rachman (1997) argues that it is these misinterpretations of the importance of one's thoughts, as well as their particular meaning about the individual, that results in a more commonplace intrusive thought developing into the full clinical manifestation observed within someone with OCD. In the same way that many of the behavioral models are predicated upon the idea of negative reinforcement occurring through compulsive behavior, many of the cognitive models of OCD are built upon the assumption that the cognitive misinterpretations present within the individual will result in resistance to one's obsessions which in turn maintains the obsessive thoughts themselves (Rachman, 1997). Still, this is not to say that the cognitive model does away with the entirety of the behavioral model's assumptions. Modern cognitive models of OCD often do not exclude all elements of behavioral theory and vice versa (Deacon & Abramowitz, 2004). Indeed, Rachman (1997; 1998) posits that exposure can be useful in clinical contexts where avoidance occurs. However, a key differentiating factor between these two models is the cognitive model assumes these misinterpretations and other cognitive mechanisms (e.g, thought-action fusion) account for the presence of obsessions and play a significant role in symptom maintenance beyond specific behavioral processes. Thus, Rachman (1997; 1998) argues that challenging the misinterpretations should be the focus of the exposure techniques being used. That is, the exposures used are done from a place of attempting to gather evidence against the obsessive thought being true rather than from a place of promoting habituation. This is not a unique conceptualization, with more modern cognitive approaches to exposure-based treatments taking a similar approach as well (e.g., Mclean et al., 2001; see Deacon & Abramowitz [2004] for a discussion of this argument and a discussion of Mclean et al., [2001]).

The variety of theories used to explain how OCD is both engendered and maintained results in these theories being both complementary amongst themselves as well as competing in other instances. This variability creates a wider, more all-encompassing understanding of OCD processes. Still, it is clear that there are challenges among these competing theories too. One particular challenge within these competing theories is the development of an understanding of the correct processes through which OCD manifests within the specific individual. Due to the variety of known factors that contribute to and often parallel OCD symptomology, exploring the relevant clinical factors in relation to OCD becomes important at the individual level. However, the heterogeneous nature of the conditions under which domain-specific symptoms develop leads to further paucity in the understanding of the contributing factors that engender OCD subtypes and related cognitions being present.

A Highly Efficacious Treatment

With the advent of cognitive-behavioral theories generally, and ERP specifically, the treatment efficacy of psychotherapy for OCD has garnered hope and symptom remission has become more common (Foa, 2010). Foa (2010) concludes that the efficacy for CBT in treating OCD, with particular emphasis on exposure-based treatments, has resulted in this treatment becoming one of the mostly widely recognized efficacious treatments for OCD. This is further reflected in the American Psychological Association's Division 12 list of empirically supported treatments for OCD currently (Society of Clinical Psychology, n.d.). In one example of the effectiveness of ERP, Franklin et al., (2000) found that ERP can reduce symptoms of OCD by up to 60%. Research has found that ERP is most effective when both exposure and response prevention are provided in tandem with one another, and some research has indicated that a mix of both in-vivo and imaginal exposure results in the greatest level of symptom reduction (Foa, 2010; Law & Boisseau, 2019) Still, many individuals do not respond to this treatment, and those that do still may have distressing symptoms present even without the same level of functional impairment or distress previously experienced (Foa, 2010). Further, when examining exposure treatments, high rates of dropout have been found to occur at times. For example, Ong et al., (2016) estimated that up to approximately 19% of individuals who started treatment did not finish.

Challenges in the Treatment of OCD

One of the primary issues within the treatment literature on OCD is that the treatments we have are often homogeneous in many respects whereas the disorder itself is heterogeneous in presentation and maintenance. For some subtypes of OCD, the majority of the treatment literature may not be as applicable as it is with regard to other subtypes. In a study of the research on the treatment of OCD, Ball et al., (1996) found that the majority of the treatment literature examined individuals who engage in compulsive cleaning or checking. This homogeneity of treatment and research when contrasted to the heterogeneity of OCD has resulted in a paucity of research examining differing treatment effects and etiological mechanisms underlying distinct subcategories of obsessive-compulsive symptom manifestations. There is, however, some evidence to indicate that differences in treatment response may vary as a function of OCD subtype. In a meta-analysis completed by Christensen et al., (1987) an emerging trend just shy of significance was identified in which those with obsessions but not compulsions may not respond as strongly to treatment generally. Similarly, Starcevic and Brakoulias (2008) further argue that symptoms consisting of obsessions but not compulsions seem to be less responsive to ERP treatment. Mataix-Cols et al., (2002) found that individuals with either hoarding symptoms or symptoms indicative of scrupulosity were more likely to either drop out of treatment or not respond to treatment as significantly, respectively. Specifically, in their research Mataix-Cols et al., (2002) found that only 21% of individuals responded to treatment who had scrupulosity symptoms as opposed to 50% of individuals whose symptoms of OCD manifested as other subtypes. Similarly, Alonso et al., (2001) found that individuals with scrupulosity experienced less symptom remission than other subtypes of OCD long-term. Still, it is not intellectually honest to say that all the research that exists supports this conclusion- that the differences in OCD subtypes will consistently result in differences in treatment outcomes. In a review of the literature, for example, Starcevic and Brakoulias (2008) describe instances in which no relationships are observed between different subtypes of OCD and treatment outcomes. Given this data, the authors conclude that treatments cannot exclusively be separated as a function of OCD subtype. However, the authors acknowledge that there is data to indicate that scrupulosity may respond differently to treatments than some other subtypes of OCD as a function of the relation of these symptoms and underlying dysfunctional cognitive styles. Based upon this finding, the authors discuss specific treatment recommendations, with one notable recommendation being the application of cognitive restructuring for scrupulosity (Starcevic & Brakoulias, 2008).

Research seems to further support the integration of varying clinical techniques with ERP and more research is finding or advocating for the importance of this process. For example, Freeston et al., (1997) examined the efficacy of CBT that combined both ERP with cognitive restructuring of four dysfunctional cognitive styles (e.g., importance of thoughts/magical thoughts, inflated responsibility, difficulty with ambiguity, and inaccurate probability) among a group of individuals with obsessions but no overt compulsions. Results indicated that the treatment was effective and symptom remission was found to have been maintained at a 6-month follow-up (Freeston et al., 1997). Similarly, Rector et al., (2019) found that integrating cognitive restructuring with ERP is an effective technique for treating OCD beyond utilizing ERP alone and Steketee et al., (2019) found that cognitive restructuring, CBT, and behavioral therapy were all effective in treating OCD. Steketee et al., (2019) further found that the behavioral interventions assessed had smaller effect sizes than the other two interventions assessed. The additive benefits and possibilities of treatment integration do not seem to exclusively extend to cognitive techniques either. Some research has found that other techniques such as acceptance and commitment therapy can also be effectively integrated with ERP (e.g., Twohig et al., 2018). Still, this does not mean the results of these studies have led to the question of whether or not additive therapy elements are consistently useful. The application of cognitive restructuring and other techniques to behavioral treatments results in a wide range of instances in which individuals will use these terms to describe varying techniques. For example, in examining the procedures for cognitive restructuring used by Freeston et al., (1997), the extent to which restructuring focused primarily on the unique cognitive mechanisms associated with OCD (e.g., responsibility of thoughts) compared to more typical techniques used in cognitive restructuring is unclear. Similarly, in examining the analyses completed by Steketee et al. (2019) it is unclear how the scope of each treatment was delineated between different researchers and treatments. Although a small detail, its importance cannot be understated. Some authors have argued for theoretical reasons why varying cognitive restructuring techniques may have potentially different outcomes clinically with regard to OCD symptom remission (e.g., Abramowitz & Jacoby, 2014). Furthermore, few studies look at specific clinical constructs in treatment as a function of OCD subtype nor personal backgrounds and experiences.

REASONS BEHIND THE HETEROGENEITY

As discussed previously, much of the existing research lumps the varying presentations of OCD that exist together in treatment research and outcomes. This is not entirely without reason. Neurologically a diagnosis of OCD can often involve the same cortical and sub-cortical structures, such as overactivation of the cortico-striatal-thalmo-cortical (CSTC) loop (Pauls et al., 2014; Stahl, 2013). Additionally, OCD generally is often shown to be related to similar deficits in neuropsychological functioning, such as executive functioning deficits (Pauls et al., 2014). However, beneath the surface of the research and hypotheses suggesting neuronal overactivation and neuropsychological deficits among those with OCD generally, there does exist some research which breaks down specific expressions of symptomology among these constructs. For instance, Nedeljkovic and colleagues (2009) found evidence of neuropsychological variability among different subtypes of OCD and nonclinical controls. The researchers found that individuals with checking compulsions performed worse than controls on a range of executive functioning tasks whereas those with washing compulsions experienced less clearly defined differences. As might be expected from these findings, it was observed that those with checking compulsions experienced deficits in their ability to recognize patterns compared to individuals with washing compulsions (Nedeljkovic et al., 2009). Similarly, Rauch and colleagues (1998) found that the severity of scrupulosity and checking compulsions was associated with increased blood flow in the striatum when compared to other symptom manifestations. In a review of the literature, Mataix-Cols et al., (2005) determined that different forms of OCD symptom expression were likely mediated by distinct neuronal processes that differ from other OCD subtypes. Therefore, these and other studies would seem to support the possibility of various neuronal and neuropsychological factors mediating genetic and environmental factors influence on symptom expressions (Mataix-Cols et al., 2005; Nedeljkovic et al, 2009; Rauch et al., 1998).

Mechanisms of Action

In the same way that there is some indication that the variability in OCD symptom expression may result in varying neuronal and neuropsychological pathways being implicated, various hypothesized mechanisms of action have been posited as possible treatment targets for those with specific subtypes of OCD. This is of particular importance in instances in which varying presentations of OCD may have different mechanisms of action. Similarly, this is vital in clinical encounters in which personal variables within a client are related to the content of their obsessions generally.

COGNITIVE AND EXPERIENTIAL MECHANISMS: RELIGIOSITY AS AN EXAMPLE

To focus on religiosity as an example of subtype differentiation within the treatment literature, a variety of studies have supported the importance of religious belief and doctrine in the etiology and maintenance of OCD symptoms (e.g., Inozu et al., 2012; Inozu et al., 2014; Mauzay & Cuttler, 2019; Mauzay et al., 2016; Williams et al., 2013). Thought-action fusion (TAF) has been found to mediate the relationships between religiosity and OCD symptoms generally (Inozu et al., 2014; Mauzay et al., 2016; Williams et al., 2013), as well as a variety of specific expressions of OCD symptomology, including washing (Inozu et al., 2014; Mauzay et al., 2016), checking (Inozu et al., 2014; Mauzay et al., 2016), neutralizing (Inozu et al., Mauzay et al., 2014), obsessing (Inozu et al., 2014; Mauzay et al., 2016), ordering (Inozu et al., 2014; Mauzay et al., 2016), and scrupulosity (Mauzay et al., 2016). At first-glance this would seem to imply the broad applicability in examining global thought-action fusion in OCD symptom presentations. As I understand it, this is a valid and clinically useful line of reasoning. However, the nuance within these studies is also important. For instance, whereas Inozu et al., (2014) examined the construct of TAF globally, Mauzay et al., (2016) and Williams et al., (2013) found differences in the mediational capabilities of TAF when the moral components of TAF were compared to that of the likelihood elements of TAF (i.e., that thoughts and actions are morally equivalent and that thoughts increase the likelihood of actions, respectively). Although Williams et al., (2013) did not break OCD down by the specific subtypes found in their measure of OCD symptoms, they found that only moral TAF was significant when looking at religious belief in the context of OCD-relevant cognitions (e.g., responsibility). Mauzay et al., (2016) independently examined moral and likelihood TAF as mediators of the relationship between religiosity and various domain-specific OCD presentations (e.g., washing, scrupulosity, checking, etc.) and found evidence supporting that there were some small differences in the mediational capabilities of moral TAF and likelihood TAF. Namely, Mauzay et al., (2016) found that moral TAF did not mediate the relationship between religiosity and ordering whereas likelihood TAF did. In contrast, both components of TAF separately were found to mediate the other subtypes of OCD symptoms assessed. Unfortunately, Mauzay et al., (2016) did not complete pairwise comparisons between these two mediators to determine the relative strength of each within each domain-specific category. The global construct of TAF as well as its specific subcategories are just one of many relevant cognitive mechanisms implicated in OCD that may vary depending on both the aspects of the mechanisms being assessed themselves as well as the domain-specific subtype of OCD examined. A variety of other dysfunctional beliefs have been implicated in OCD too (e.g., perfectionism and certainty [PC], responsibility and threat estimation [RT], and importance and need to control thoughts [ICT]; OCCWG, 1997; OCCWG, 2005) and have been found to mediate these relationships (e.g., Inozu et al., 2012; Mauzay & Cuttler, 2019). The OCCWG (1997; 2005) identified these constructs after extensive research on the cognitive factors related to OCD. Inozu et al., (2012) found that ICT and RT mediate the relationships between religiosity and OCD. Similarly, Mauzay and Cuttler (2019) found that these same two mediators mediated the relationship between religiosity and scrupulosity. However, in contrast to Inozu et al., (2012), Mauzay and Cuttler (2019) found that all three dysfunctional beliefs (i.e., ICT, RT, and PC) mediated the relationships between religiosity and OCD generally. Mauzay and Cuttler (2019) further found that the relationships between paranormal beliefs and both overall OCD and scrupulosity specifically were mediated by these same mechanisms. Differences between the relative strength of these different mediators were also observed within the varying mediation analyses conducted by Mauzay and Cuttler (2019) which suggests there may be variability among the relevance of each dysfunctional belief clinically depending on either the belief system and/or the manifestation of OCD assessed.

THE ROLE OF TRAUMA AND OTHER PSYCHOLOGICAL CONSTRUCTS IN THE ETIOLOGY OF OCD

Other constructs that are not based within religious thought nor related to specific cognitive mechanisms are also clear areas of relevance in clinical settings for their possible etiological significance in OCD. Past instances of trauma have been implicated in the potential outcome of OCD symptom manifestation and have been shown to be prevalent among those with OCD. Specifically, it has been found that up to 54% of individuals diagnosed with OCD will endorse a past traumatic experience (Cromer et al., 2007). Cromer et al. (2007) further found that obsessions and checking, as well as symmetry and ordering, were associated with past trauma endorsement in contrast to contamination and cleaning subtypes. In a recent study, Barzilay et al. (2019) found that trauma experiences were associated with OCD symptomology generally among a youth sample. Notably, Barzilay and colleagues (2019) found that this association was particularly strong among domain-specific symptoms that were generally indicative of scrupulosity. Furthermore, the same aforementioned cognitive mechanisms have been found to be possible etiological mechanisms in these relationships. Indeed, Briggs and Price (2009) found that the dysfunctional beliefs discussed previously mediated the relationship between childhood trauma exposure and OCD symptoms. Similar patterns of different psychological constructs being relevant to the partial or full manifestation of specific OCD subtypes have also been observed as well, such as disgust sensitivity (Inozu et al., 2014), anger (Piacentino et al., 2016), shame (Szentágotai-Tâtar et al., 2020), fear (Piacentino et al., 2016), and impulsivity (Piacentino et al., 2016).

IMPLEMENTATION WITHIN A TREATMENT CONTEXT

Taken as a whole, it seems highly likely that different mechanisms and experiences may engender different OCD symptoms. As such, further attention to the specific application of treatment options for the differing constructs (e.g., moral TAF, intolerance of ambiguity, religiosity, trauma history, shame, etc.) is a vital step for the field of mental health so as to continue to develop more effective treatment interventions. What is now becoming clearer is the importance of and need to begin integrating these constructs explicitly within the established treatment regimen of ERP and other forms of treatment. Lopatka and Rachman (1995) argue that responsibility of thoughts/actions are a fundamental etiological factor in OCD as demonstrated by these authors having found that when decreasing this cognitive construct OCD symptoms decrease as well. Lopatka and Rachman (1995) are not the only researchers to have articulated this, as can be seen in Briggs and Price (2009) as well as Diedrich et al. (2016). Research has even gone so far as to determine that the presence of these dysfunctional cognitive styles predict the later development of OCD symptom manifestation when controlling for prior psychopathology (Abramowitz et al., 2006).

Working with Religiosity

Religious obsessions have been conceptualized as likely developing from a stricter system of religious belief as well as a conceptual understanding of belief that is more focused on negative religious ideology (e.g., punishment; Abramowitz & Jacoby, 2014; Rachman, 1997; Rachman, 1998). As such, an important question for a clinician in working with OCD through an ERP framework may be how this individual may grow both spiritually as well as through symptom change? In working with individuals with OCD it has been argued that challenging negative appraisals related to obsessive content in the same way as you would other diagnoses may only result in brief symptom remission and could potentially result in negative reinforcement (Abramowitz & Jacoby, 2014). Instead, in these instances a clinician must focus on attending to the underlying mechanisms that are at play through assisting a client in engaging in cognitive restructuring. In examining intolerance of ambiguity as an example, this can be done through assisting the client in restructuring their thoughts through the lens of learning to be able to tolerate the ambiguity present within their obsessions (Abramowitz & Jacoby, 2014; Grayson, 2010). This is of particular importance within scrupulosity given that many of the obsessions in relation to religious thought and doctrine will be inherently ambiguous, with uncertainty being a matter of fact rather than preference (Abramowitz & Jacoby, 2014). I work through this with clients by exploring their disquiet regarding the desire to determine something is impossible when at most it can only be improbable. Personally, I have found great success in working with clients to examine the origins of their need for certainty, as well as other cognitive mechanisms, and exploring the extent to which this original messaging is relevant to their life now/their obsessions. Another activity I have found useful is inviting my clients to engage in a dialogue with themselves in which they determine if their feared obsessions must be addressed or if God will simply be able to understand their OCD. Similarly, discussing the difference between obsessions and sin can also be useful in sessions depending on the client (Abramowitz & Jacoby, 2014). The basis of these discussions is predicated upon the agreement between client and clinician about the impossibility of certainty which allows for a wide avenue of therapeutic dialogue to take place (Grayson, 2010).

Abramowitz and Jacoby (2014) outline the lack of trust clients with scrupulosity often have in their own religious doctrine and describe treatment being framed as a way in which clients can pursue their faith more fully. This is important in treating those with scrupulosity. This dichotomy of positive and negative religious coping when juxtaposed with their relevance in a client's life mirrors the same pattern described by Beck (2011) in which an individual examines negative experiences in a way that is consistent with previously constructed maladaptive schemata while simultaneously not attending to information countering this same belief. I believe that attending to this discrepancy can be a powerful tool in exploring the ways in which a client wants to relate to their own conceptual understanding of God (or their object/individual of worship) and their belief system. In working with clients, I often invite them to discuss with me the ways in which their current beliefs and cognitive appraisals may serve them and the ways in which they may be causing them to pull away from what ideally should be a meaningful and valued aspect of their life. Similar to what is discussed here, Abramowitz and Jacoby (2014) have further identified a number of ways in which the contrast between an individual's obsessions and their personal faith can be dealt with. Specifically, the authors posit that addressing the cognitive mechanism of difficulty with ambiguity can be accomplished through approaching the necessity of ambiguity as a necessity of faith. That is, assisting the individual in understanding that part of their growth in their own faith can occur through learning to tolerate and accept the ambiguity present within their feared religious obsessions and compulsions (Abramowitz & Jacoby, 2014).

In looking at the research available, it is clear that varying cognitive mechanisms are more or less relevant in differing subtypes of OCD (e.g., Inozu et al., 2012; Mauzay et al., 2016; Mauzay & Cuttler, 2019). Therefore, addressing a specific mechanism of action is not a necessary step, and indeed may detract from treatment, in every case example of an individual with OCD. Rather than having a strict rule-bound way to implement these techniques into the overall treatment of ERP, it becomes important for a clinician to use clinical judgment within their own cases to develop a way of determining the relevant mechanisms to treat. This can be done through administering questionnaires, such as the Obsessional Beliefs Questionnaire (OCCWG, 1997; OCCWG, 2005), to develop a starting point in treatment, but can also be as complex as co-creating an understanding of the mechanisms present within the client at the outset of therapy. I often co-create the cognitive mechanisms through which clients view their OCD as having manifested. This is accomplished through addressing the specific, idiosyncratic experiences my clients have had and exploring in what ways they see this as informing their current personal conditional beliefs/intermediate beliefs in the present. As the term conditional beliefs implies, this is where more traditional cognitive therapy techniques can be useful in the treatment of OCD.

Conditional and intermediate beliefs compromise a category of beliefs an individual can have that play a role in eliciting automatic thoughts (Beck, 2011). For the purposes of my use of the term in the present writing, I am primarily referring to rules and assumptions an individual may be making about their OCD or the factors related to said disorder (Beck, 2011). Thus, rather than relying exclusively on the current mechanisms identified by researchers and groups such as the OCCWG (1997; 2005), I believe it is imperative to assist the client in creating their own narrative for how they have come to understand the world and how this understanding may influence how they think about their obsessions. It seems simplistic to assume that all of the cognitive mechanisms that have been identified are the relevant constructs in these relationships. Even more so, I think it is simplistic to reify these constructs and declare them to be the most important. And lastly, although I think the benefits of this research lay an excellent foundation on which we need to build from, using the specific dysfunctional beliefs previously identified should not take the place of the development of idiosyncratic treatment approaches to understanding the individual's personal cognitive processes- as these may be consistent with the research or entirely contradictory to it. As this last point emphasizes, I am in agreement with Norcross and Wampold (2011; 2018) as well as Yalom (2002) who advocate for the co-creative and individualized nature of psychotherapy for each individual. This is not contradictory towards utilizing empirical evidence to justify specific treatment decisions. In fact, this is what I consider to be an important part of utilizing the available evidence. That is, utilizing the empirical foundation of a psychotherapy while creating the unique treatment approach I develop with my clients that is tailored to the individual is grounded in an evidence base (e.g., Norcross & Wampold, 2011). Thus, although I appreciate that Freeston et al., (1997) explored the underlying cognitive mechanisms within one's OCD symptoms, I also think that in addition to targeting these mechanisms of action an idiosyncratic approach to developing unique cognitive mechanisms can also be necessary at the individual level.

For example, there have been instances where incredibly idiosyncratic mechanisms have engendered OCD. An example in which this seemed to have occurred was when an individual seeking help for OCD symptoms was not obsessive regarding blasphemous religious thoughts themselves. Instead, the individual had begun to obsess about the possibility that in having the thought that they would like to "go to hell" or "sell" their soul they may have accidently spoken it aloud so quietly that, although it was unable to be heard by the individual themselves, an accidental "agreement" or "transaction" took place to the extent that they are no longer able to enter heaven upon their death. In examples such as this it is clear that some cognitive mechanisms are at play, though this hardly would fit with any of the previously described cognitive mechanisms developed by the OCCWG (1997; 2005) given that it is the fear that in having the thought they may accidently "speak" at an imperceivable level. Thus, the implicated mechanism is the belief that these thoughts will result in spoken words occurring which will result in an individual giving up their soul because it was spoken aloud. Regardless of the inherent irrationality of this it may be hard for someone with OCD to work through this thought pattern in an effort to promote logic, which is why authors such as Abramowitz and Jacoby (2014) do not advocate for this treatment strategy. Furthermore, as well be discussed in the next section, in doing so (i.e., examining the lack of logic behind this obsession) one is always at the risk of engaging in culturally incompetent practice. Therefore, developing unique ways to target idiosyncratic mechanisms becomes important because an individual's OCD symptoms often are unique to the person. In this example, it took for the individual to critically look at their religious doctrine and determine the extent to which they believe God would allow them to "burn in hell" for these perceived transgressions, coupled with exposure and response prevention promoting both habituation as well as an increased tolerance of ambiguity, for symptom remission to occur.

Cultural Humility in Examining Cognitive Mechanisms of Action

A fundamental aspect of the cognitive work described in the present writing is the cultural humility it allows for a clinician to hold when working with their clients. It is important to address the cognitive mediators previously discussed so as to pursue further symptom remission, but also has been argued as being relevant for promoting cultural sensitivity and humility in treatment by various authors (e.g., Mauzay et al., 2016). It is easy to find ways in which one's personal religious convictions could feel attacked through treatment rather than the underlying mechanisms that may have instilled OCD symptoms. Thus, the strategies described in which cognitive mediators are challenged avoids doing this through addressing mechanisms of action among religious and spiritual clients instead (Mauzay et al., 2016). This involves challenging assumptions a client might have about their ability to deal with the ambiguity or the adaptive versus maladaptive elements related to thought-action fusion (Abramowitz & Jacoby, 2014). Notably, this does not involve telling someone that these beliefs are maladaptive themselves, but instead helping them explore in what ways applying these cognitive mechanisms to their fears and daily life may no longer be serving a functional purpose. This is articulated by Abramowitz and Jacoby (2014) as being a necessary element of effective exposure in the therapy process because it allows the person to understand that they can tolerate their obsessions rather than merely habituating to them. With scrupulosity, this also has a dual benefit given that matters of religious faith are inherently complex in that it can be hard to ever know with certainty (Abramowitz & Jacoby, 2014).

Trauma and OCD

As mentioned previously, a large portion of individuals with OCD report having experienced a trauma in the past (Cromer et al., 2007) and trauma can have an influence on the types of symptoms of OCD engendered (Barizilay et al., 2019). Rachman (2010) argues for the relevance of betrayal among those with OCD and provides examples of individuals with OCD who articulate specific instances of betrayal within their life having influenced their symptoms. Additionally, researchers have argued that traumatic experiences can result in the same cognitive mechanisms developing that were previously discussed (Briggs & Price, 2009). Thus, a thorough assessment of both a client's trauma as well as the role in which their traumatic history parallels or engenders their OCD symptoms is of paramount importance clinically (Dykshoorn, 2014). This does not necessarily require specific separate clinical tasks to be accomplished. Instead, it can be utilized through an increased appreciation and understanding of the role of trauma in OCD symptom maintenance. I have found that this can be easily implemented through attending to the rules and conditional beliefs commonly explored among empirically supported treatments for PTSD (e.g., cognitive processing therapy; Resick et al., 2016) and their relation to the presence of obsessions and compulsions within an individual with OCD.

Values as They Relate to Obsessive Content

Previous theorists and clinicians have supported claims indicating that an individual's personal values influence feared obsessive content among individuals with OCD. As discussed by Abramowitz and Jacoby (2014) as well as Rachman (2003), it is likely that an individual who has intrusive thoughts about a topic has strong values associated with the presence of these obsessions. That is, an individual who has intrusive thoughts of assaulting their grandmother often may be distressed by this precisely because they are a loving, caring grandchild. This is based within the cognitive theory of obsessions. Namely, that one's obsessions results in negative appraisals about what these obsessions say about the individual (Abramowitz & Jacoby, 2014; Rachman, 2003). Although this fact is painful for the individual struggling with OCD, it opens up a wide array of treatment avenues. Working towards discussing personal religious values within faith, as was discussed in the previous section of the current writing, is relevant here too (Abramowitz & Jacoby, 2014). Further, so too is a more general exploration of this linking of personal values and OCD content and subtypes. For example, working with a client towards exploring what it might mean about them that they are worried about hurting a loved one through asking questions such as if this implies that they value the individual rather than their desire to act upon these fears? This is also an instance where exposure can be very powerful in sessions. I have worked with individuals who feared hurting me in sessions before (i.e., aggressive obsessions) and often am willing to engage in exposure exercises where it is clear that I personally trust that they have no intention of harming me. I have seen this work therapeutically through what I consider to be two pathways- through both general patterns of ERP which allows us to test the individual's obsessions as well as through this providing an experience through which the individual understands that others (i.e., me) do not view them as "sick" or defective in some way. Notably, care should be taken so as to not repetitively repeat this conversation with those with OCD, however, as this may result in decreased treatment effectiveness (Foa et al., 2012; Yadin et al., 2012).

Emotional Change Processes

Although the focus of the present writing has been on the cognitive mechanisms that engender and maintain OCD, with a particular emphasis on scrupulosity, it is important to point out that emotional change processes have been implicated within OCD as well. As mentioned previously, these include examples such as anger (Piacentino et al., 2016) and disgust sensitivity (Inozu et al., 2014). Furthermore, emotional change processes can also be argued to play a fundamental role in the processes through which shifts in cognitive mechanisms occur. Interestingly, when looking at the manualized treatment of ERP few components of the treatment are devoted specifically to the application of cognitive restructuring (Foa et al., 2012; Yadin et al., 2012). Similarly, even fewer emotional processes within the treatment of OCD are acknowledged (Foa et al., 2012; Yadin et al., 2012). The broad, though not complete, separation of cognitive and affective treatments within the field of psychotherapy among some clinicians is unfortunate in more ways than one. As Greenberg (2008) points out, the schemas individuals develop are often highly integrated to the extent they consist of both cognitive and affective structures. Although the bidirectional relationship between cognition and emotion appears to be clear, many clinicians may focus on one at the expense of the other. In the same way I believe more cognitive techniques should be incorporated into ERP, I too think that focus on the affectively laden schemata an individual holds is important clinically. At the heart of psychotherapy, the importance of meaning construction has often been identified and emotion is believed to play a large role in this process (Greenberg, 2008). Moreover, emotion has been articulated as being an important context through which effective cognitive restructuring can occur (e.g., Safran & Greenberg, 1982). Therefore, I believe that focusing on the experiential change processes within the treatment of OCD is vital for effective treatment to take place. This position is supported by recent research indicating that transdiagnostic emotion-focused treatments are an effective way of treating OCD (Shaw et al., 2020). Safran and Segal (1990) argue for the relevance of working with emotional immediacy and emotional presence throughout the restructuring process. I often will explore the underlying emotional dissonance that may be present within someone with OCD (e.g., their desire to care for a sick family member but subsequent obsessions of hurting them, or someone's desire to practice their religious beliefs comfortably but avoidance of said practices) and work towards having these two "sides" speak to one another through chair exercises or cognitive techniques.

Therefore, I see techniques like the two-chair technique for a self-evaluative split (Greenberg et al., 1993) as putting two appraisals or other cognitive mechanisms against one another similarly to how a cognitive therapist might have an individual examine their thoughts from an attorney's perspective or role play two sides of a thought in an effort to determine a thoughts legitimacy and make new meaning from the situation (Leahy, 2003). I view these techniques as different ways of going about providing clients with a means of shifting their cognitive framework, all of which require a skilled application of giving a "voice" to two sides of one's appraisals in an effort to more formally examine its meaning. The important difference in applying these techniques to OCD is to keep in mind any possible negative reinforcement that may be occurring through cognitive restructuring and ensuring that an individual is not utilizing it in a maladaptive way (Abramowitz & Jacoby, 2014; Foa et al., 2012; Yadin et al., 2012).

As discussed in a previous section, these techniques being utilized in sessions are compatible with also implementing standard ERP treatment. ERP and other forms of CBT do not need to be utilized in contrast to these techniques and instead can easily complement one another (see Safran & Segal [1990] for an excellent discussion of interpersonal and emotional processes and the relevance of them from within a CBT framework). Moreover, although the possible integration of acceptance, values clarification, cognitive restructuring, and attention to emotion are not clearly articulated within some of the treatment manuals for ERP, other work by Foa and Wilson (2001) on treating OCD through ERP clearly identifies instances in which some of these processes can directly or indirectly be useful. Many individuals who use manuals become aware through their use of a manual that doing so does not necessitate a rigid, prescriptive approach to the session structure (Forbat et al., 2016; Mansfield & Addis, 2001). It is worth noting that knowing manuals can be applied flexibly increases clinician willingness to consider manuals which further supports reasoning as to why increased flexibility with the use of manuals is important (Addis & Krasnow, 2000; Mansfield & Addis, 2001).

CONCLUSION

As has been discussed throughout this chapter, the importance of varying cognitive and emotional constructs as well as related experiences within an individual with OCD is garnering increased attention in the research literature. It is my hope that this chapter can serve as one of many calls to action within our field to take this emerging literature seriously so as to promote increased treatment efficacy for those suffering from OCD. Moreover, continuing to apply varying techniques within the gold-standard of ERP treatment for OCD is becoming increasingly important and may result in both increased treatment efficacy as well as increased treatment palatability and cultural humility (e.g., Abramowitz & Jacoby, 2014; Freeston et al., 1997; Mauzay et al., 2016). There is growing evidence that varying clinical and individual constructs may result in an individual being predisposed towards developing OCD generally, as well as certain subtypes specifically (e.g., Abramowitz et al., 2006; Inozu et al., 2012; Mauzay and Cuttler, 2019). Thus, the presence of these varying mechanisms of action, such as the previously described dysfunctional beliefs, may be indicative of particular subtypes of OCD having developed or developing in the future (e.g., Abramowitz et al., 2006; Inozu et al., 2012; Mauzay and Cuttler, 2019). Increased research and clinical attention must continue to be given to these areas so as to support continued growth within the field of mental health. Moreover, it is clear that targeting these cognitive constructs for treatment is becoming progressively recognized as a vital skill to utilize when treating someone with OCD (Diedrich et al., 2016; Lopatka & Rachman, 1995).

REFERENCES

Abramowitz, J. S., & Jacoby, R. J. (2014). Scrupulosity: A cognitive-behavioral analysis and implications for treatment. *Journal of*

Obsessive-compulsive and Related Disorders, 3, 140-149. doi: http://dx.doi.org/10/1016/j.jocrd.2013.12.007.

Abramowitz, J. S., Khandker, M., Nelson, C. A., Deacon, B. J., & Rygwall, R. (2006). The role of cognitive factors in the pathogenesis of obsessive-compulsive symptoms: A prospective study. *Behaviour Research and Therapy*, 44, 1361-1374. doi: 10.1016/j.brat.2005.09.011.

Addis, M. E., & Krasnow, A. D. (2000). A national survey of practicing psychologists' attitudes toward psychotherapy treatment manuals. *Journal of Consulting and Clinical Psychology*, 68, 331-339.

Alonso, P., Menchon, J. M., Pifarre, J., Mataix-Cols, D., Torres, L., Salgado, P., & Vallejo, J. (2001). Long-term follow-up and predictors of clinical outcome in obsessive-compulsive patients treated with serotonin reuptake inhibitors and behavioral therapy. *Journal of Clinical Psychiatry*, 62, 535-540. doi: 10.408/jcp.v62n07a06.

American Psychiatric Association. (2013). *Diagnostic and statistical manual of mental disorders* (5th ed.). American Psychiatric Publishing.

Ball, S. G., Baer, L., & Otto, M. W. (1996). Symptom subtypes of obsessive-compulsive disorder in behavioral treatment studies: A quantitative Review. *Behaviour Research and Therapy,* 34, 47-51.

Barzilay, R., Patrick, A., Calkins, M. E., Moore, T. M., Gur, R. C., & Gur, R. E. (2019). Associations between early-life trauma and obsessive compulsive symptoms in community youth. *Depression and Anxiety*, 36, 586-595. doi: 10.1002/da.22907.

Beck, J. S. (2011). *Cognitive behavior therapy: Basics and beyond* (2nd ed.). Guilford Press.

Briggs, E. S., & Price, I. R. (2009). The relationship between adverse childhood experience and obsessive-compulsive symptoms and beliefs: The role of anxiety, depression, and experiential avoidance. *Journal of Anxiety disorders*, 23, 1037-1046. doi: 10.1016/j.janxdis.2009.07.004.

Cassin, S. E., & Rector, N. A. (2012). Psychological Models of Obsessive-Compulsive and Spectrum Disorders: From Psychoanalytic to Behavioral Conceptualizations. In Steketee, G. (Ed.), *The Oxford Handbook of Obsessive compulsive and Spectrum Disorders*. (pp. 209-232). Oxford University Press.

Christensen, H., Hadzi-Pavlovic, D., Andrews, G., & Mattick, R. (1987). Behavior therapy and tricyclic medication in the treatment of obsessive-compulsive disorder: A quantitative review. *Journal of Consulting and Clinical Psychology*, 55, 701-711. doi: https://doi.org/10.1037/0022-006X.55.5.701.

Cromer, K. R., Schmidt, N. B., & Murphy, D. L. (2007). An investigation of traumatic life events and obsessive-compulsive disorder. *Behaviour Research and Therapy*, 45, 1683-1691. doi: 10.1016/j.brat.2006.08.018.

Deacon, B. J., & Abramowitz, J. S. (2004). Cognitive and behavioral treatments for anxiety disorders: A review of the meta-analytic findings. *Journal of Clinical Psychology*, 60, 429-441. doi: 10.1002/jclp.10255.

Diedrich, A., Sckopke, P., Schwartz, C., Schlegl, S., Osen, B., Stierle, C., & Voderholzer, U. (2016). Change in obsessive beliefs as predictor and mediator of symptom change during treatment of obsessive-compulsive disorder – a process-outcome study. *BMC Psychiatry*, 16, 1-10. doi: 10.1186/s12888-016-0914-6.

Dykshoorn, K. (2014). Trauma-related obsessive-compulsive disorder: A review. *Health Psychology and Behavior Medicine*, 2, 517-528. doi: http://dx.doi.org/10.1080/21642850.2014.905207.

Foa, E. (2010). Cognitive behavioral therapy of obsessive-compulsive disorder. *Dialogues in Clinical Neuroscience*, 12, 199-207. doi: 10.31887/DCNS.2010.12.12.2/efoa.

Foa, E. B., & Wilson, R. (2001) *Stop obsessing: How to overcome your obsessions and compulsions* (2 ed.). Bantam Books.

Foa, E. B., Yadin, E., & Lichner, T. K. (2012). *Exposure and response (ritual) prevention for obsessive-compulsive disorder: Therapist Guide* (2 ed.). Oxford University Press.

Forbat, L., Black, L., & Duglar, K. (2016). What clinicians think of manualized psychotherapy interventions: Findings from a systematic review. *Journal of Family Therapy*, 37, 409-428. doi: https://doi.org/10.1111/1467-6427.12036.

Franklin, M. E., Abramowitz, J. S., Kozak, M. J., Levitt, J. T., & Foa, E. B. (2000). Effectiveness of exposure and ritual prevention for obsessive-compulsive disorder: Randomized compared with nonrandomized samples. *Journal of Consulting and Clinical Psychology*, 68, 594-602. doi: 10.1037//0022-006X.68.4.594.

Freeston, M. H., Ladouceur, R., Gagnon, F., Thibodeau, N., Rhéaume, J., Letarte, H., & Bujold, A. (1997). Cognitive-behavioral treatment of obsessive-thoughts: A controlled study. *Journal of Consulting and Clinical Psychology*, 65, 405-413. doi: 10.1037/0022-006X.65.3.405.

Grayson, J. B. (2010). OCD and intolerance of uncertainty: Treatment issues. *Journal of Cognitive Psychotherapy: An International Quarterly*, 24, 3-15. doi: 10.1891/0889-8391.24.1.3.

Greenberg, L. (2008). Emotion and cognition in psychotherapy: The transforming power of affect. *Canadian Psychology*, 49, 49-59. doi: 10.1037/0708-5591.49.1.49.

Greenberg, L. S., Rice, L. N., & Elliott, R. (1993). *Facilitating emotional change: The moment-by-moment process*. Guilford Press.

Inozu, M., Karanci, A. N., & Clark, D. A. (2012). Why are religious individuals more obsessional? The role of mental control beliefs and guilt in Muslims and Christians. *Journal of Behavior Therapy and Experimental Psychiatry*, 43, 959-966. doi:10.1016/j.jbtep.2012.02.004.

Inozu, M., Ulukut, F. O., Ergun, G., & Alcolado, G. M. (2014). The mediating role of disgust sensitivity and thought-action fusion between religiosity and obsessive compulsive symptoms. *International Journal of Psychology*, 49, 334-341. doi:10.1002/ijop.12041.

Law, C., & Boisseau, C. L. (2019). Exposure and response prevention in the treatment of obsessive-compulsive disorder: Current perspectives. *Psychology Research and Behavior Management*, 12, 1167-1174.

Leahy, R. L. (2003). *Cognitive therapy techniques: A practitioner's guide*. New York, NY: Guilford Press.

Lochner, C., Hemmings, S. M. J., Kinnear, C. J., Nel, D., Hemmings, S. M. J., Seedat, S., Moolman-Smook, J. C., & Stein, D. J. (2008). Cluster analysis of obsessive-compulsive symptomology: Identifying obsessive-compulsive disorder subtypes. *Israel Journal of Psychiatry and Related Science*, 45, 164-176.

Lopatka, C., & Rachman, S. (1995). Perceived responsibility and compulsive checking: An experimental analysis. *Behaviour Research and Therapy*, 33, 673-684. doi: 10.1016/0005-7967(94)00089-3.

Mansfield, A. K., & Addis, M. E. (2001). Manual-based psychotherapies in clinical practice part 1: Assets, liabilities, and obstacle to dissemination. *Evidence Based Mental Health*, 4, 68-69.

Mataix-Cols, D., Marks, I. M., Greist, J. H., Kobak, K. A., & Baer, L. (2002). Obsessive-compulsive symptoms dimensions as predictors of compliance with and response to behaviour therapy: Results from a controlled trial. *Psychotherapy and Psychosomatics*, 71, 255-262. doi: 10.1159/0000664812.

Mataix-Cols, D., Rosario-Campos, M. C. D., & Leckman, J. F. (2005). A multidimensional model of obsessive-compulsive disorder. *American Journal of Psychiatry*, 162, 228-238. doi: 10.1176/appi.ajp.162.2.228.

Mauzay, D., Spradlin, A., & Cuttler, C. (2016). Devils, Witches, and Psychics.: The role of thought-action fusion in the relationships between obsessive-compulsive features, religiosity, and paranormal beliefs. *Journal of Obsessive-Compulsive and Related Disorders*, 11, 113-120. doi: https://doi.org/10/1016/j.jocrd.2016.10.003.

Mauzay, D., & Cuttler, C. (2019). Dysfunctional cognitions mediate the relationships between religiosity, paranormal beliefs, and symptoms of obsessive-compulsive disorder. *Mental Health, Religion, and Culture*, 21, 838-850. doi: https://doi.org/10.1080/13674676.2019.1583176.

Mclean, P. D., Whittal, M. L., Thordarson, D. S., Taylor, S., Söchting, I., Koch, W. J., Paterson, R., & Anderson, K. W. (2001). Cognitive versus behavior therapy in the group treatment of obsessive-compulsive disorder. *Journal of Consulting and Clinical Psychology*, 69, 205-214.

Nedeljkovic, M., Kyrios, M., Moulding, R., Doron, G., Wainwright, K., Pantelis, C., Purcell, R., & Maruff, P. (2009). Differences in neuropsychological performance between subtypes of obsessive-compulsive disorder. *Australian and New Zealand Journal of Psychiatry*, 43, 216-226.

Norcross, J. C., & Wampold, B. E. (2011). What works for whom: Tailoring psychotherapy to the person. *Journal of Clinical Psychology: In Session*, 67, 127-132. doi: 10.1002/jclp.20764.

Norcross, J. C., & Wampold, B. E. (2018). A new therapy for each patient: Evidence-based relationships and responsiveness. *Journal of Clinical Psychology*, 74, 1889-1906.

Obsessive Compulsive Cognitions Working Group. (1997). Cognitive assessment of obsessive-compulsive disorder. *Behaviour Research and Therapy*, 35, 667-681. doi:10.1016/S0005-7967(97)00017-X.

Obsessive Compulsive Cognitions Working Group. (2005). Psychometric validation of the obsessive belief questionnaire and interpretation of intrusions inventory- Part 2: Factor analyses and testing of a brief version. *Behaviour Research and Therapy*, 43, 1527-1542. doi:10.1016/j.brat.2004.07.010.

Ong, C. W., Clyde, J. W., Bluett, E. J., Levin, M. E., & Twohig, M. P. (2016). Dropout rates in exposure with response prevention for obsessive-compulsive disorder: What do the data really say? *Journal of Anxiety Disorders*, 40, 8-17. doi: 10.1016/j.janxdis.2016.03.006.

Pauls, D. L., Abramovitch, A., Rauch, S. L., & Geller, D. A. (2014). Obsessive-compulsive disorder: An integrative genetic and neurobiological perspective. *Nature Reviews, Neuroscience*, 15, 410-424. doi: 10.1038/nrn3746.

Piacentino, D., Pasquini, M., Tarsitani, L., Berardelli, I., Roselli, V., Maraone, A., & Biondi, M. (2016). The association of anger with symptom subtypes in severe obsessive-compulsive disorder outpatients. *Psychopathology*, 49, 40-46. doi: https://doi.org/10.1159/000443900.

Rachman, S. (1997). A cognitive theory of obsessions. *Behaviour Research and Therapy*, 35, 793-802.

Rachman, S. (1998). A cognitive theory of obsessions: Elaborations. *Behaviour Research and Therapy*, 36, 385-401.

Rachman, S. (2003). *The Treatment of Obsessions*. Oxford University Press.

Rachman, S. (2010). Betrayal: A psychological analysis. *Behaviour Research and Therapy*, 48, 304-311. doi: https://doi.org/10.1016/j.brat.2009.12.002.

Rauch, S. L., Dougherty, D. D., Shin, L. M., Alpert, N. M., Manzo, P., Leahy, L., Fischman, A. J., Jenike, M. A., & Baer, L. (1998). Neural correlates of factor-analyzed OCD symptom dimensions: A PET study. *CNS Spectrums*, 3, 37-43. doi: https://doi.org/10.1017/S1092852900006167.

Resick, P. A., Monson, C. M., & Chard, K. M. (2016). *Cognitive processing therapy for PTSD: A Comprehensive manual*. Guilford Press.

Rector, N. A., Richter, M. A., Katz, D., & Leybman, M. (2019). Does the addition of cognitive therapy for exposure and response prevention for obsessive compulsive disorder enhance clinical efficacy? A randomized controlled trial in a community setting. *British Journal of clinical Psychology*, 58, 1-18. doi: 10.1111/bjc.12188.

Safran, J. D., & Greenberg, L. S. (1982). Eliciting "hot cognitions" in cognitive behaviour therapy: Rationale and Procedural Guidelines. *Canadian Psychology*, 23, 83-87. 10.1037/h0081247.

Safran, J. D., & Segal, Z. V. (1990). *Interpersonal process in cognitive therapy*. Basic Books.

Schalkwyk, G. I. V., Bhalla, I. P., Griepp, M., Kelmendi, B., Davidson, L., & Pittenger, C. (2016). Toward understanding the heterogeneity in obsessive-compulsive disorder: Evidence from narratives in adult patients. *Australian and New Zealand Journal of Psychiatry*, 50, 74-81. doi: https://doi.org/10.1177/0004867415579919.

Shaw, A. M., Halliday, E. R., & Ehrenreich-May, J. (2020). The effect of transdiagnostic emotion-focused treatment on obsessive-compulsive symptoms in children and adolescents. *Journal of Obsessive-Compulsive and Related Disorders*, 26, 1-11. doi: https://doi.org/10.1016/j.jocrd.2020.100552.

Society of Clinical Psychology. (n.d.). Psychological Treatments. Retrieved from https://www.div12.org/treatments/.

Stahl, S. M. (2013). *Stahl's essential psychopharmacology: Neuroscientific basis and practical applications* (4th ed.). Cambridge University Press.

Starcevic, V., & Brakoulias, V. (2008). Symptom subtypes of obsessive-compulsive disorder: Are they relevant for treatment? *Australian and New Zealand Journal of Psychiatry*, 42, 651-661. doi:10.1080/00048670802203442.

Steketee, G., Siev, J., Yovel, I., Lit, K., & Wilhelm, S. (2019). Predictors and moderators of cognitive and behavioral therapy outcomes for OCD: A patient-level mega-analysis of eight sites. *Behavior Therapy*, 50, 165-176. doi: 10.1016/j.beth.2018.04.004.

Szentágotai-Tâtar, A., Nechita, D., & Miu, A. C. (2020). Shame in anxiety and obsessive-compulsive disorders. *Current Psychiatry Reports*, 22, 14-16. doi:https://doi.org/10/1007/s11920-1142-9.

Twohig, M. P., Abramowitz, J. S., Smith, B. M., Fabricant, L. E., Jacoby, R. J., Morrison, K. L., Bluett, E. J., Reuman, L., & Blakey, S. M. (2018). Adding acceptance and commitment therapy to exposure and response prevention for obsessive-compulsive disorder: A randomized controlled trial. *Behaviour Research and Therapy*, 108, 1-9. doi: 10.1016/j.brat.2018.06.005.

Williams, A. D., Lau, G., & Grisham, J. R. (2013). Though-action fusion as a mediator of religiosity and obsessive-compulsive symptoms. *Journal of Behavior Therapy and Experimental Psychiatry*, 44, 207-212. doi: https://dx.doi/org/10/1016/j.jbtep.2012.09.004.

Yadin, E., Foa., E. B., & Lichner, T. K. (2012). *Treating your OCD with exposure and response (ritual) prevention: Workbook* (2nd Ed.). Oxford University Press.

Yalom, I. (2002). *The gift of therapy: An open letter to a new generation of therapists and their patients* (7th ed.). HarperCollins.

In: Obsessive-Compulsive Disorder
Editor: Jeffrey L. Nelson
ISBN: 978-1-68507-310-7
© 2021 Nova Science Publishers, Inc.

Chapter 3

ACUTE-ONSET SUBTYPES OF PEDIATRIC OBSESSIVE-COMPULSIVE DISORDER: PEDIATRIC ACUTE-ONSET NEUROPSYCHIATRIC SYNDROME AND PEDIATRIC AUTOIMMUNE NEUROPSYCHIATRIC DISORDERS ASSOCIATED WITH STREPTOCOCCAL INFECTIONS

Canan Kuygun Karci[*], MD*
Department of Child and Adolescent Psychiatry,
Dr. Ekrem Tok Psychiatry Hospital, Adana, Turkey

---

[*] Corresponding Author's E-mail: c_kuy@hotmail.com.

ABSTRACT

Pediatric acute-onset neuropsychiatric syndrome (PANS) and pediatric autoimmune neuropsychiatric disorders associated with streptococcal infections (PANDAS) are acute-onset subtypes of obsessive-compulsive disorder (OCD) in children. PANDAS include sudden-onset OCD symptoms and new-onset tics due to streptococcal infection. PANDAS were first defined by Swedo in 1998. In 2012, a new diagnostic criterion (PANS) was proposed for patients who met all PANDAS criteria except for association with streptococcal infection. For the diagnosis of PANS, sudden-onset OCD symptoms and/or severe food restriction are accompanied by at least two of the following: depression/emotional lability, anxiety, irritability, aggression and/or oppositional behavior, behavioral regression, somatic symptoms, deteriorated school performance, and sensorimotor abnormalities required. Although it is hypothesized that the pathogenesis of PANDAS and Sydenham's chorea is similar, definitive proof of the pathogenesis is lacking. Also, there are many unresolved questions about diagnostic criteria and the clinical approach for PANS/PANDAS. This creates confusion and difficulty in treatment and follow-up. In this chapter, the diagnostic criteria, clinical aspects, and current treatment approaches of PANDAS and PANS will be discussed.

INTRODUCTION

The age of onset of obsessive-compulsive disorder (OCD) has a bimodal distribution with one peak in pre-adolescence childhood and another in adulthood. There is increasing evidence that the immune system plays a role in the pathophysiology of OCD (Marazziti, Mucci and Fontenelle 2018). In childhood, OCD and tics may develop after an immune response with group A Streptococci (GAS) infection. GAS is one of the most common agents in childhood bacterial infections (Soderholm et al., 2017). However, the absence of OCD or tics in all children with GAS infections seems to be related to individual predispositions (Murphy, Sajid and Goodman 2006).

OCD and/or tics triggered by GAS infections are defined as pediatric autoimmune neuropsychiatric disorders associated with streptococcal infections (PANDAS) (Swedo et al., 1998). GAS infections can be detected in nearly 30% of cases of PANDAS (Leon et al., 2018). To show a relationship with GAS infection, there should be GAS colonization in throat culture and/or elevation in antistreptolysin-O (ASO) or antiDNase B levels (Johnson et al., 2010). Although there may not be an increase in ASO and antiDNase B levels due to GAS infections, it is also possible that the levels of these antibodies may remain high for months after infection. Therefore, it is difficult to definitively show the relationship between GAS infections and symptom exacerbations of PANDAS.

In 2012, a broader category was defined: the presence of acute-onset OCD and/or restricted food intake and that did not require association with GAS infection; pediatric acute-onset neuropsychiatric syndrome (PANS) (Swedo, Leckman and Rose 2012). Studies have reported that both PANS and PANDAS symptom exacerbations may occur due to other bacterial or viral infections and psychosocial stress (Thienemann et al., 2017, Lehman et al., 2018, Katz 2019). Lack of definitive proof on the pathophysiology, and unresolved questions about the diagnostic criteria and clinical approach bring great challenges for both physicians and patients (Orlovska et al., 2017). In this chapter, PANS and PANDAS will be examined in view of the current literature data.

DIAGNOSTIC CRITERIA

The definition of PANDAS was first made in 1998 with 50 patients that presented sudden-onset OCD or tic disorder symptoms after GAS infection (Swedo et al., 1998) (Table 1). The number of cases meeting the diagnostic criteria for PANDAS is relatively low because it is difficult to show the temporal association between the onset or exacerbation of OCD and/or tic symptoms and GAS infection (Gabbay et al., 2008). In addition, it is often difficult to interpret acute-onset symptoms triggered by non-GAS infections (Kurlan, Johnson and Kaplan 2008).

To resolve the confusion and controversy arising from these reasons, a new broader diagnostic label (PANS) was proposed in 2012. For the diagnosis of PANS, sudden-onset OCD symptoms and/or severe food restriction are accompanied by at least two of the following: depression/emotional lability, anxiety, irritability, aggression and/or oppositional behavior, behavioral regression, somatic symptoms, deteriorated school performance, and sensorimotor abnormalities required (Table 1) (Swedo, Leckman and Rose 2012). Unlike PANDAS, whereas tic disorder, prepubertal onset, and association with GAS infection are not required for the diagnosis of PANS, sudden-onset OCD and restricted food intake are prerequisites for PANS.

Table 1. Diagnostic criteria of PANDAS and PANS

PANDAS	PANS
1. Presence of diagnosis of OCD and/or tic disorder	1. Abrupt, dramatic onset of obsessive-compulsive disorder or severely restricted food intake (<48 h).
2. Pediatric onset (symptoms first evident between age 3 years and beginning of puberty)	2. Concurrent and severely acute onset of at least two of the following symptoms:
3. Episodic course (characterized by abrupt onset of symptoms or dramatic symptom exacerbations)	a. Anxiety b. Emotional lability and/or depression c. Irritability, aggression, and/or severely oppositional behaviors
4. Association with group A beta-hemolytic streptococcus infection	d. Behavioral (developmental) regression e. Deterioration in school performance f. Sensorimotor abnormalities g. Somatic signs or symptoms, including sleep disturbances, enuresis or urinary frequency.
5. Association with neurologic abnormalities (motoric hyperactivity and adventitious movements including choreiform movements or tics).	3. Symptoms are not better explained by a known neurologic or medical disorder, such as Sydenham chorea, systemic lupus erythematosus, Tourette syndrome or others.

OCD: Obsessive-compulsive disorder, PANDAS: pediatric autoimmune neuropsychiatric disorders associated with streptococcal infections, PANS: Pediatric acute-onset neuropsychiatric syndrome.

Pathophysiology

It has been suggested that the pathophysiology of Sydenham chorea (SC) and PANDAS, which have similar neuropsychiatric symptoms and etiologic agents, may also be similar. It is thought that autoantibodies against streptococcal proteins that specifically target proteins, especially in the basal ganglia, play a major role in the pathophysiology of PANDAS, as in SC (Cunningham 2016). These cross-reactions mostly occur between streptococcal N-acetyl-beta-D-glucosamine and neuronal lysoganglioside and tubulin (Murphy, Kurlan and Kaplan 2010, Cunningham 2014). This results in receptor dysregulation, disruptions in the cortex-basal ganglia circuit, and neuroinflammation (Kumar, Wiiliams and Chugani 2015, Cunningham and Cox 2016).

Anti-basal ganglia antibodies were found to be higher in patients with post-streptococcal neuropsychiatric symptoms and movement disorders (SC and PANDAS) compared with healthy controls (Church et al., 2002, Church, Dale and Giovannoni 2004). In the literature, studies are showing the presence of antibodies against dopamine receptor (D1 and D2), pyruvate kinase, beta-tubulin and lysoganglioside-GM1, and increased calcium calmodulin-dependent kinase II activity (CaMKII-activity) in patients with PANDAS (Pavone et al., 2004, Kirvan et al., 2006, da Rocha, Correa and Teixeira 2008, Baj et al., 2020, Shimasaki et al., 2020). However, there are also studies reporting that these antibodies are not discriminative for the diagnosis of PANS or PANDAS (Singer et al., 2005, Brilot et al., 2011, Hesselmark and Bejerot 2017).

Autoimmune or inflammatory diseases are detected at a higher rate both in patients with PANS/PANDAS and their relatives than in healthy controls or children with OCD (Stagi et al., 2014, Jaspers-Fayers et al., 2017, Gromark et al., 2019), which supports the view that there is a role of inflammation and/or immune mechanisms in the pathophysiology of PANS/PANDAS.

Previous studies have shown the relationship between the neuroinflammatory process and NADPH oxidase-2 (NOX2) activation, lipopolysaccharide (LPS), and oxidative stress (Sorce and Krause 2009,

Cahill-Smith and Li 2014, Zhao, Jaber and Lukiw 2017, Loffredo et al., 2020a). Based on this, a recent study investigated the relationship between PANDAS and oxidative stress (Loffredo et al., 2020b). It was reported that serum NOX2, LPS, and isoprostane levels were elevated in children with PANDAS, confirming the link between increased oxidative stress and neuropsychiatric manifestations of PANDAS. In addition, it has been suggested that serum zonulin levels are also high, which increases gut permeability and is the reason for the high serum LPS level (Loffredo et al., 2020b). Recently, the possible role of gut microbiota in the pathophysiology of PANDAS has also attracted attention. In the study of Quagliariello et al., (2020), it was determined that there were changes in the gut microbiota of children with PANS/PANDAS. Vitamin D deficiency (Celik et al., 2016, Stagi et al., 2018) and the presence of a polymorphism in the mannose-binding lectin gene, which plays a role in the immune response (Celik et al., 2018), are other topics investigated in patients with PANDAS.

CLINICAL ASPECTS

Patients with PANS/PANDAS are thought to have a more severe and disruptive onset and clinical course, require more urgent evaluation and have a greater family impact than in children with OCD (Jaspers-Fayer et al., 2017). PANS/PANDAS is more common in males and the age of onset is earlier than pediatric OCD (Swedo, Leckman and Rose 2012, Murphy et al., 2015, Gromark et al., 2019).

The onset of symptoms is gradual in typical OCD, by contrast, PANS/PANDAS is characterized by the abrupt onset or exacerbation of OCD symptoms. Although 'sudden-onset' is among the diagnostic criteria, in a study of 47 patients with PANS, only 19 had acute-onset symptoms (Frankovich et al., 2015). In PANDAS, there should be 6 months between a GAS infection and the onset of OCD or tic disorder, and 6 weeks between neuropsychiatric exacerbations and GAS infections (Swedo et al., 1998). However, there are conflicting findings in the literature regarding the temporal relationship between GAS infections and neuropsychiatric exacerbations in PANDAS (Nielsen et al., 2019).

Few studies have shown a relevant decline in school performance, hand-writing difficulties, and impairment in neuropsychologic functions such as visuospatial skills, attention, elaboration speed, short memory tasks, and recall in patients with PANS/PANDAS (Murphy et al., 2015, Gamucci et al., 2019, Lepri et al., 2019, Colvin et al., 2021). The most common neurologic impairments in PANDAS are hyperactivity and choreiform movements or tics, which should be differentiated from SC. Choreiform movements, like those in SC, are observed in almost 30% of patients with OCD and PANDAS (Baj et al., 2020). By contrast, OCD, emotional lability, and anxiety may accompany SC (Punukollu et al., 2016). However, OCD in SC is much more severe and is accompanied by hypotonic chorea (Crealey et al., 2015). There are also differences in the clinical course of the two disorders. SC is a monophasic disorder that mostly results in remission, whereas PANDAS is recurrent and chronic (Orefici et al., 2016).

In a longitudinal study, it was shown that 72% of children with PANDAS experienced at least one exacerbation of symptoms during the follow-up, 12% showed clinically significant OCD symptoms, and 88% had complete or near-complete remission after a mean of 3.3 years (Leon et al., 2018). During the follow-up period, 33% of the patients had at least one psychiatric comorbid diagnosis, and the most common diagnosis was attention-deficit/hyperactivity disorder (ADHD).

In a PANS follow-up study, although complete remission was not achieved, a significant improvement was observed in the symptoms of 85% of patients after a mean 3 years of follow-up (Gromark et al., 2021). A new psychiatric diagnosis was added to 38% of the patients during the follow-up period and ADHD was the most frequent diagnosis. More thyroid abnormalities (anti-TPO, TSH, T4) and elevation of tumor necrosis factor (TNF)-alpha and interleukin 1-beta were detected in patients with PANS during follow-up compared with baseline. In this study, it was reported that earlier onset, more functional impairment, and more autoimmune or inflammatory comorbidities were observed in patients with PANS with a chronic course. It was observed that somatic symptoms such as pain, enuresis, and skin rashes observed in patients with PANS became rare in the follow-up (Gromark et al., 2019, Gromark et al., 2021).

TREATMENT

PANS/PANDAS treatment guidelines were developed by the PANS/PANDAS Research Consortium and published in the special issue of the Journal of Child and Adolescent Psychopharmacology in 2017. In this guideline, treatment recommendations are grouped under 3 headings:[1]

- Antimicrobials and secondary prophylaxis
- Immunomodulatory therapies
- Symptom management through cognitive behavior therapy (CBT) and psychiatric medication use.

Antimicrobials and Secondary Prophylaxis

The most common infections associated with PANS and PANDAS are upper respiratory tract infections such as pharyngitis, rhinitis, and sinusitis; the most common microbiomes are GAS, Mycoplasma pneumonia, and influenza. In addition, asymptomatic pharyngeal GAS may also be associated with PANS/PANDAS. Penicillin (10 days), amoxicillin (10 days) or benzathine penicillin G (once) is recommended for primary antimicrobial therapy in cases of PANS/PANDAS associated with GAS infection, and azithromycin (5 days), cephalexin (10 days), cefadroxil (10 days), clindamycin (10 days) or clarithromycin (10 days)

---

[1] https://www.pandasppn.org/guidelines.

are recommended if penicillin allergy is present. Similarly, initiation of GAS treatment is recommended in patients with non-streptococcal PANS whose association with GAS infection cannot be demonstrated. Amoxicillin-clavulanate is recommended for rhinosinusitis, annual influenza vaccine is recommended for influenza, and macrolides, azithromycin or tetracycline are recommended for mycoplasma pneumonia (Cooperstock et al., 2017).

In a randomized, double-blind, placebo-controlled study, a greater improvement in OCD symptoms was observed in the group treated with azithromycin for 4 weeks compared with the group receiving placebo (Murphy et al., 2017). In a large survey study, it was reported that antibiotic treatment given in patients with PANS was effective at a rate of 8-52% (Calaprice, Tona and Murphy 2017).

In one study, antibiotic prophylaxis was not found to be superior to placebo in preventing GAS infection and symptom exacerbation (Garvey et al., 1999), whereas, in another study without a placebo control, antibiotic prophylaxis was found to be effective (Snider et al., 2005). In a large cohort study, patients with PANS and PANDAS continued prophylaxis with benzathine benzylpenicillin every 21 days for at least 5 years after treatment with amoxicillin-clavulanate for 10 days to 3 weeks. Significant clinical improvement was observed in 75% of patients with PANDAS in 3-5 months and 88.4% of patients with PANS in 6-12 months. In addition, long-term antibiotic prophylaxis has been shown to prevent recurrence of neurologic symptoms in more than half of patients with PANS and PANDAS (Lepri et al., 2019). The Consortium also recommends antibiotic prophylaxis for at least 1 or 2 years for children who are most severely affected and with multiple neuropsychiatric exacerbations associated with GAS (Cooperstock et al., 2017).

Tonsillectomy has also been considered as an option in the treatment of PANDAS. Two observational studies are reporting no relationship between tonsillectomy and symptom severity (Murphy et al., 2013, Pavone et al., 2014). In addition, tonsillectomy was considered effective in case series (Demesh, Virbalas and Bent 2015). Data on the effect of tonsillectomy in PANDAS are very limited because there is no prospective, controlled study.

Due to the possible role of gut microbiota in the pathophysiology of PANS/PANDAS, probiotics were thought to have a place in the treatment, but there is no evidence that they were effective. Based on its relationship with immune regulatory mechanisms, vitamin D3 supplementation is recommended for patients with PANS to keep the serum 25-hydroxy vitamin D level above 30 ng/mL (Cooperstock et al., 2017).

Immunomodulatory Therapies

Immunomodulatory treatment recommendations in patients with PANS/PANDAS are as follows:

- Mild to moderate flare: non-steroidal anti-inflammatory drugs (NSAIDs) (such as ibuprofen, naproxen, sulindac, celecoxib), if no improvement corticosteroids are recommended.
- Moderate to severe flare: prednisone, dexamethasone pulse, intravenous (IV) methylprednisolone or intravenous immunoglobulin (IVIG)
- Severe to extreme flare: dexamethasone pulse, IV methylprednisolone; therapeutic plasma exchange (TPE) is recommended in the presence of life-threatening disease. If TPE is not available IVIG is recommended (Frankovich et al., 2017).

There are case reports or case series showing improvement in PANS/PANDAS symptoms and neuroinflammation with immunomodulatory treatments (Frankovich et al., 2015, Kovacevic, Grand and Swedo 2015, Kumar, Wiiliams and Chugani 2015, Brown et al., 2017). Evidence on the effect of TPE and IVIG treatment on improvement is insufficient. Although improvement has been reported in case reports or case series, the results of randomized controlled trials and survey studies do not provide strong evidence to support the use of TPE or IVIG (Sigra, Hesselmark and Bejerot 2018).

The response with NSAIDs in PANS/PANDAS has been reported in case reports or case series (Sigra, Hesselmark and Bejerot 2018). In an observational study, it was found that the duration of symptom exacerbation was shortened with both prophylactic and early use (<4 weeks) of NSAIDs (Spartz et al., 2017). It is also necessary to be careful in terms of adverse effects related to NSAIDs. Similar to NSAIDs, it has been reported that the use of corticosteroids, especially in recent-onset cases and in the early period (flares >14 days), is effective in symptom remission and shortens the exacerbation period (Frankovich et al., 2017, Sigra, Hesselmark and Bejerot 2018). There are also no controlled, prospective studies for the use of corticosteroids. In addition, the presence of infection should be excluded when starting corticosteroid therapy and it should be kept in mind that corticosteroids may exacerbate some psychiatric symptoms.

Psychoactive Drugs and CBT

The effectiveness of CBT in pediatric OCD is well established. Although the efficacy of CBT alone in patients with PANS/PANDAS has not been investigated in randomized controlled trials, two uncontrolled studies reported remission of OCD symptoms with CBT + antibiotic therapy (Nadeau et al., 2015) and CBT + selective serotonin reuptake inhibitor (SSRI) (Storch et al., 2006).

SSRIs with proven efficacy in pediatric OCD has not been investigated in controlled and systematic studies in PANS/PANDAS. Efficacy and adverse effects have been reported in case reports of the use of antibiotics, immunomodulators or other psychotropic drugs in combination with SSRIs (Sigra, Hesselmark and Bejerot 2018). It has been emphasized that there may be periodic changes in the treatments because both OCD and other accompanying psychiatric symptoms in

PANS/PANDAS can change through the course of the disease (Thienemann et al., 2017).

In the literature, studies are reporting that antibiotic treatment and/or prophylaxis are more effective in patients with PANS/PANDAS instead of psychiatric treatments (Mahapatra, Panda and Sagar 2017, Hesselmark and Bejerot 2019), as well as publications reporting that psychiatric treatment provides an improvement in PANS/PANDAS, similarly in pediatric OCD (Wilbur et al., 2019).

Drugs with proven efficacy in pediatric OCD and CBT are very likely to also be effective in PANS/PANDAS. However, immune and inflammatory processes are receiving greater attention among researchers.

Conclusion

Although studies on PANS/PANDAS have increased, the evidence value is still low and confusing points remain in the majority. Most of the data in the literature come from case reports or case series. In systematic studies, samples were often too small or there was no comparison group, or PANS/PANDAS was compared with movement disorders, tic disorders or OCD. Prospective, randomized controlled studies with larger samples are needed.

Determining the predisposing factors, supporting the diagnostic criteria with laboratory or imaging findings, and having more evidence-based information about exacerbations and the clinical course will also help clarify the treatment algorithm.

References

Baj J., Sitarz E., Forma A., Wróblewska K., Karakuła-Juchnowicz H. 2020. Alterations in the Nervous System and Gut Microbiota after β-

Hemolytic Streptococcus Group A Infection-Characteristics and Diagnostic Criteria of PANDAS Recognition. *Int J Mol Sci.* Feb 21;21(4):1476. doi: https://10.3390/ijms21041476. PMID: 32098238; PMCID: PMC7073132.

Brilot F., Merheb V., Ding A., Murphy T., Dale RC.2011. Antibody binding to neuronal surface in Sydenham chorea, but not in PANDAS or Tourette syndrome. *Neurology;* 76(17):1508-13.

Brown K. D., Farmer C., Freeman G. M. Jr., Spartz J. E., Farhadian B., Thienemann M., Frankovich J. 2017. Effect of early and prophylactic nonsteroidal anti-inflammatory drugs on flare duration in pediatric acute-onset neuropsychiatric syndrome: An observational study of patients followed by an academic community-based pediatric acute-onset neuropsychiatric syndrome clinic. *J Child Adolesc Psychopharmacol*; 27(7):619-28.

Cahill-Smith S., Li J. M. 2014. Oxidative stress, redox signalling and endothelial dysfunction in ageing-related neurodegenerative diseases: a role of NADPH oxidase 2. *Br J Clin Pharmacol*; 78(3):441-53.

Calaprice D., Tona J., Murphy T. K. 2017. Treatment of Pediatric Acute-Onset Neuropsychiatric Disorder in a Large Survey Population. *J Child Adolesc Psychopharmacol.* doi: https://10.1089/cap.2017.0101. PubMed PMID:28832181.

Celik G. G., Tas D. A., Tahiroglu A. Y., Erken E., Seydaoglu G., Ray P. C., Avci A. 2018. Mannose-Binding Lectin2 gene polymorphism in PANDAS patients. *Noro Psikiyatri Arsivi,* 56, 99-105.

Celik G., Tas D., Tahiroglu A., Avci A., Yuksel B., Cam P. 2016. Vitamin D deficiency in obsessive-compulsive disorder patients with pediatric autoimmune neuropsychiatric disorders associated with streptococcal infections: A case control study. *Noro Psikiyatri Arsivi*, 53, 31-34.

Church A. J., Cardoso F., Dale R. C., Lees A. J., Thompson E. J., Giovannoni G. 2002 Antibasal ganglia antibodies in acute and persistent Sydenham's chorea. *Neurology*; 59(2):227-31.

Church A. J., Dale R. C., Giovannoni G. 2004. Anti-basal ganglia antibodies: A possible diagnostic utility in idiopathic movement disorders? *Arch. Dis. Child,* 89, 611-614.

Colvin M. K., Erwin S., Alluri P. R., Laffer A., Pasquariello K., Williams K. A. 2021. Cognitive, Graphomotor, and Psychosocial Challenges in Pediatric Autoimmune Neuropsychiatric Disorders Associated With Streptococcal Infections (PANDAS). *J Neuropsychiatry Clin Neurosci;* 33(2):90-97. doi: https://10.1176/appi.neuropsych. 20030065. Epub 2020 Dec 2. PMID: 33261524.

Cooperstock M. S., Susan E. Swedo, Mark S. Pasternack, Tanya K. 2017. Murphy, and for the PANS/PANDAS Consortium. *Journal of Child and Adolescent Psychopharmacology.* 594-606. http://doi.org/10. 1089/cap.2016.0151.

Crealey M., Allen N. M., Webb D., Bouldin A., Sweeney N. M., Peake D., Tirupathi S., Butler K., King M. D. 2015. Sydenhams chorea: Not gone but perhaps forgotten. *Arch. Dis. Child,* 100, 1160-1162.

Cunningham M. W. 2014. Rheumatic fever revisited. *Nat. Rev. Cardiol,* 11, 123.

Cunningham M. W. 2016. Post-streptococcal autoimmune sequelae: Rheumatic fever and beyond. In: *Streptococcus pyogenes: Basic Biology to Clinical Manifestations.* Edited by Ferretti J. J., Stevens D. L., Fischetti V. A. Oklahoma City (OK), University of Oklahoma Health Sciences Center.

Cunningham M. W., Cox C. J. 2016. Autoimmunity against dopamine receptors in neuropsychiatric and movement disorders: a review of Sydenham chorea and beyond. *Acta Physiol* (Oxford). 216(1):90-100.

da Rocha F. F., Correa H., Teixeira A. L. 2008 Obsessive-compulsive disorder and immunology: A review. *Prog. Neuro Psychopharmacol. Biol. Psychiatry,* 32, 1139-1146.

Demesh D., Virbalas J. M., Bent J. P. 2015. The role of tonsillectomy in the treatment of pediatric autoimmune neuropsychiatric disorders associated with streptococcal infections (PANDAS). *JAMA Otolaryngol Head Neck Surg;* 141(3):272-5. doi: https://10.1001/ jamaoto.2014.3407. PubMed PMID: 25569020

Frankovich J., Susan Swedo, Tanya Murphy, Russell C. Dale, Dritan Agalliu, Kyle Williams, Michael Daines, Mady Hornig, Harry Chugani, Terence Sanger, Eyal Muscal, Mark Pasternack, Michael Cooperstock, Hayley Gans, Yujuan Zhang, Madeleine Cunningham, Gail Bernstein, Reuven Bromberg, Theresa Willett, Kayla Brown, Bahare Farhadian, Kiki Chang, Daniel Geller, Joseph Hernandez, Janell Sherr, Richard Shaw, Elizabeth Latimer, James Leckman, Margo Thienemann, and PANS/PANDAS Consortium. 2017. *Journal of Child and Adolescent Psychopharmacology.* 574-593. http://doi.org/10.1089/cap.2016.0148.

Frankovich J., Thienemann M., Pearlstein J., Crable A., Brown K., Chang K. 2015. Multidisciplinary clinic dedicated to treating youth with pediatric acute-onset neuropsychiatric syndrome: Presenting characteristics of the first 47 consecutive patients. *J Child Adolesc Psychopharmacol* 2015;25(1):38-47.

Gabbay V., Coffey B. J., Babb J. S., Meyer L., Wachtel C., Anam S., Rabinovitz B. 2008. Pediatric autoimmune neuropsychiatric disorders associated with streptococcus: Comparison of diagnosis and treatment in the community and at a specialty clinic. *Pediatrics* 122:273-278.

Gamucci A., Uccella S., Sciarretta L., D'Apruzzo M., Calevo M. G., Mancardi M. M., Veneselli E., De Grandis E. 2019 PANDAS and PANS: Clinical, Neuropsychological, and Biological Characterization of a Monocentric Series of Patients and Proposal for a Diagnostic Protocol. *J Child Adolesc Psychopharmacol.* 29(4):305-312. doi: https://10.1089/cap.2018.0087. Epub 2019 Feb 6. PMID: 30724577.

Garvey M. A., Perlmutter S. J., Allen A. J., Hamburger S., Lougee L., Leonard H. L., Witowski M. E., Dubbert B., Swedo S. E. 1999. A pilot study of penicillin prophylaxis for neuropsychiatric exacerbations triggered by streptococcal infections. *Biol Psychiatry.* 45(12):1564-71. PubMed PMID: 10376116.

Gromark C., Harris R. A., Wickstr M. R., Horne A., Silverberg-Mörse M., Serlachius E., Mataix-Cols D. 2019. Establishing a pediatric acute-onset neuropsychiatric syndrome clinic: baseline clinical features of the pediatric acute-onset neuropsychiatric syndrome cohort at Karolinska Institutet. *J Child Adolesc Psychopharmacol* 29(8):625-633.

Gromark C., Hesselmark E., Djupedal I. G., Silverberg M., Horne A., Harris R. A., Serlachius E., Mataix-Cols D. 2021. A Two-to-Five Year Follow-Up of a Pediatric Acute-Onset Neuropsychiatric Syndrome Cohort. *Child Psychiatry Hum Dev*. 1-11. doi: https://10.1007/s10578-021-01135-4. Epub ahead of print. PMID: 33559023; PMCID: PMC7870456.

Hesselmark E., Bejerot S. 2017. Biomarkers for diagnosis of pediatric acute neuropsychiatric syndrome (PANS) - sensitivity and specificity of the Cunningham panel. *J Neuroimmunol*. 312:31-7.

Hesselmark E., Bejerot S. 2019. Patient Satisfaction and Treatments Offered to Swedish Patients with Suspected Pediatric Acute-Onset Neuropsychiatric Syndrome and Pediatric Autoimmune Neuropsychiatric Disorders Associated with Streptococcal Infections. *J. Child Adolesc. Psychopharmacol*. 29, 634-641.

Jaspers-Fayer F., Han S. H. J., Chan E., McKenney K., Simpson A., Boyle A., Ellwyn R., Stewart S. E. 2017. Prevalence of Acute-Onset Subtypes in Pediatric Obsessive-Compulsive Disorder. *J Child Adolesc Psychopharmacol*. 27(4):332-341. doi: https://10.1089/cap.2016.0031. Epub 2017 Jan 25. PMID: 28121463.

Johnson D. R., Kurlan R., Leckman J., Kaplan E. L. 2010. The Human Immune Response to Streptococcal Extracellular Antigens: Clinical, Diagnostic, and Potential Pathogenetic Implications. *Clinical Infectious Diseases*. 50(4):481-490. PubMed PMID: 20067422.

Katz B. Z. 2019. Streptococcal Infections and Exacerbations in Pediatric Autoimmune Neuropsychiatric Disorder Associated With Streptococcal Infection: A Systematic Review and Meta-Analysis. Pediatr. *Infect. Dis. J*. 38, e190-e191.

Kirvan C. A., Swedo S. E., Snider L. A., Cunningham M. W. 2006. Antibody-mediated neuronal cell signaling in behavior and movement disorders. *J. Neuroimmunol*. 179, 173-179.

Kovacevic M., Grant P., Swedo S. E. 2015. Use of intravenous immunoglobulin in the treatment of twelve youths with pediatric autoimmune neuropsychiatric disorders associated with streptococcal infections. *J Child Adolesc Psychopharmacol* 25(1):65-9.

Kumar A., Williams M. T., Chugani H. T. 2015. Evaluation of basal ganglia and thalamic inflammation in children with pediatric autoimmune neuropsychiatric disorders associated with streptococcal infection and Tourette syndrome: a positron emission tomographic (PET) study using 11C-[R]PK11195. *J Child Neurol.* 30(6):749-56.

Kurlan R., Johnson D., Kaplan E. L. 2008. Streptococcal infection and exacerbations of childhood tics and obsessive-compulsive symptoms: A prospective blinded cohort study. *Pediatrics* 121:1188-1197.

Lehman M., Navarro V., Suchecki D., Handa R. 2018. Introduction to the PANS special issue. *J. Neuroendocrinol.* 30, 12612.

Leon J., Hommer R., Grant P., Farmer C., D'Souza P., Kessler R., Williams K., Leckman J. F., Swedo S. 2018. Longitudinal outcomes of children with pediatric autoimmune neuropsychiatric disorder associated with streptococcal infections (PANDAS). *Eur Child Adolesc Psychiatry.* 27(5):637-643. doi: https://10.1007/s00787-017-1077-9. Epub 2017 Nov 8. PMID: 29119300.

Lepri G., Rigante D., Bellando Randone S., Meini A., Ferrari A., Tarantino G., Cunningham M. W., Falcini F. 2019. Clinical-Serological Characterization and Treatment Outcome of a Large Cohort of Italian Children with Pediatric Autoimmune Neuropsychiatric Disorder Associated with Streptococcal Infection and Pediatric Acute Neuropsychiatric Syndrome. *J Child Adolesc Psychopharmacol.* 29(8):608-614. doi: https://10.1089/cap.2018.0151. Epub 2019 May 29. PMID: 31140830.

Loffredo L., Ettorre E., Zicari A. M., Inghilleri M., Nocella C., Perri L., Spalice A., Fossati C., De Lucia M. C., Pigozzi F., Cacciafesta M., Violi F., Carnevale R. 2020a. Oxidative stress and gut-derived lipopolysaccharides in neurodegenerative disease: role of NOX2. *Oxidative Med Cell Longev.* 8630275.

Loffredo L., Spalice A., Salvatori F., De Castro G., Guido C. A., Zicari A. M., Ciacci P., Battaglia S., Brindisi G., Ettorre E., Nocella C., Salvatori G., Duse M., Violi F., Carnevale R. 2020b. Oxidative stress and gut-derived lipopolysaccharides in children affected by paediatric autoimmune neuropsychiatric disorders associated with streptococcal infections. *BMC Pediatr.* 20(1):127. doi: https://10.1186/s12887-020-02026-8. PMID: 32188439; PMCID: PMC7079429.

Mahapatra A., Panda P. K., Sagar R. 2017. Pediatric autoimmune neuropsychiatric disorders associated with streptococcal infection treated successfully with a course of oral antibiotics. *Asian J. Psychiatr.* 25, 256-257.

Marazziti D., Mucci F., Fontenelle L. F. 2018. Immune system and obsessive-compulsive disorder. *Psychoneuroendocrinology.* 93:39-44. doi: https://10.1016/j.psyneuen.2018.04.013. Epub 2018 Apr 13. PMID: 29689421.

Murphy T. K., Brennan E. M., Johnco C., Parker-Athill E. C., Miladinovic B., Storch E. A., Lewin A. B. 2017. A double-blind randomized placebo-controlled pilot study of azithromycin in youth with acute-onset obsessive-compulsive disorder. *J Child Adolesc Psychopharmacol.* 27(7):640-51.

Murphy T. K., Kurlan R., Leckman J. 2010. The immunobiology of Tourette's disorder, pediatric autoimmune neuropsychiatric disorders associated with Streptococcus, and related disorders: a way forward. *J Child Adolesc Psychopharmacol.* 20(4):317-31.

Murphy T. K., Lewin A. B., Parker-Athill E. C., Storch E. A., Mutch P. J. 2013. Tonsillectomies and adenoidectomies do not prevent the onset of pediatric autoimmune neuropsychiatric disorder associated with group A streptococcus. *Pediatr Infect Dis J.* 32(8):834-8. doi: https://10.1097/INF.0b013e31829062e2. PubMed PMID: 23518825; PubMed Central PMCID: PMCPMC3740796.

Murphy T. K., Patel P. D., McGuire J. F., Kennel A., Mutch P. J., Parker-Athill E. C., Hanks C. E., Lewin A. B., Storch E. A., Toufexis M. D., Dadlani G. H., Rodriguez C. A. 2015. Characterization of the pediatric acuteonset neuropsychiatric syndrome phenotype. *J Child Adolesc Psychopharmacol* 25:14-25.

Murphy T. K., Sajid M. W., Goodman W. K. 2006. Immunology of obsessive-compulsive disorder. *Psychiatr. Clin. North Am.* 29, 445-469.

Nadeau J. M., Jordan C., Selles R. R., Wu M. S., King M. A., Patel P. D., Hanks C. E., Arnold E. B., Lewin A. B., Murphy T. K., Storch E. A. 2015. A pilot trial of cognitive-behavioral therapy augmentation of antibiotic treatment in youth with pediatric acute-onset neuropsychiatric syndrome-related obsessive-compulsive disorder. *J Child Adolesc Psychopharmacol.* 25(4):337-43.

Nielsen M. Ø., Köhler-Forsberg O., Hjorthøj C., Benros M. E., Nordentoft M., Orlovska-Waast S. 2019. Streptococcal Infections and Exacerbations in PANDAS: A Systematic Review and Meta-analysis. *Pediatr Infect Dis J.* 38(2):189-194. doi: https://10.1097/INF.0000000000002218. PMID: 30325890.

Orefici G., Cardona F., Cox C. J., Cunningham M. W. 2016. Pediatric Autoimmune Neuropsychiatric Disorders Associated with Streptococcal Infections (PANDAS). In: Ferretti J. J., Stevens D. L., Fischetti V. A., editors. *Streptococcus pyogenes: Basic Biology to Clinical Manifestations [Internet]*. Oklahoma City (OK): University of Oklahoma Health Sciences Center; 2016-. PMID: 26866234.

Orlovska S., Vestergaard C. H., Bech B. H., Nordentoft M., Vestergaard M., Benros M. E. 2017. Association of streptococcal throat infection with mental disorders: Testing key aspects of the PANDAS hypothesis in a nationwide study. *JAMA Psychiatry.* 74(7):740-6.

Pavone P., Bianchini R., Parano E., Incorpora G., Rizzo R., Mazzone L., Trifiletti R. R. 2004. Anti-brain antibodies in PANDAS versus uncomplicated streptococcal infection. *Pediatr Neurol.* 30(2):107-10.

Pavone P., Rapisarda V., Serra A., Nicita F., Spalice A., Parano E., Rizzo R., Maiolino L., Mauro P. D., Vitaliti G., Coco A., Falsaperla P., Trifiletti R. R., Cocuzza S. 2014. Pediatric autoimmune neuropsychiatric disorder associated with group a streptococcal infection: the role of surgical treatment. *Int J Immunopathol*

Pharmacol. 27(3):371-8. doi: https://10.1177/039463201402700307. PubMed PMID: 25280028.

Punukollu M., Mushet N., Linney M., Hennessy C., Morton M. 2016. Neuropsychiatric manifestations of Sydenham's chorea: A systematic review. *Dev Med Child Neurol* 58:16-28.

Quagliariello A., Del Chierico F., Russo A., Reddel S., Conte G., Lopetuso L. R., Ianiro G., Dallapiccola B., Cardona F., Gasbarrini A., Putignani L. 2018. Gut microbiota profiling and gut-brain crosstalk in children affected by pediatric acute-onset neuropsychiatric syndrome and pediatric autoimmune neuropsychiatric disorders associated with streptococcal infections. *Front. Microbiol.* 9, 1-15.

Shimasaki C., Frye R. E., Trifiletti R., Cooperstock M., Kaplan G., Melamed I., Greenberg R., Katz A., Fier E., Kem D., Traver D., Dempsey T., Latimer M. E., Cross A., Dunn J. P., Bentley R., Alvarez K., Reim S., Appleman J. 2020. Evaluation of the Cunningham Panel™ in pediatric autoimmune neuropsychiatric disorder associated with streptococcal infection (PANDAS) and pediatric acute-onset neuropsychiatric syndrome (PANS): Changes in antineuronal antibody titers parallel changes in patient symptoms. *J Neuroimmunol.* 15; 339:577138. doi: https://10.1016/j.jneuroim. 2019.577138. Epub 2019 Dec 15. PMID: 31884258.

Sigra S., Hesselmark E., Bejerot S. 2018. Treatment of PANDAS and PANS: a systematic review. *Neurosci Biobehav Rev.* 86:51-65. doi: https://10.1016/j.neubiorev.2018.01.001. Epub 2018 Jan 6. PMID: 29309797.

Singer H. S., Hong J. J., Yoon D. Y., Williams P. N. 2005. Serum autoantibodies do not differentiate PANDAS and Tourette syndrome from controls. *Neurology.* 65(11):1701-7.

Snider L. A., Lougee L., Slattery M., Grant P., Swedo S. E. 2005. Antibiotic prophylaxis with azithromycin or penicillin for childhood-onset neuropsychiatric disorders. *Biol Psychiatry.* 57(7):788-92. doi: https://10.1016/j.biopsych.2004.12.035. PubMed PMID: 15820236.

Soderholm A. T., Barnett Timothy C., Sweet Matthew J., Walker Mark J. 2017. Group a streptococcal pharyngitis: Immune responses involved in bacterial clearance and GAS-associated immunopathologies. *Journal of Leukocyte Biology.* 103, 193-213. doi: https://10.1189/jlb. 4MR0617-227RR.

Sorce S., Krause K. H. 2009. NOX enzymes in the central nervous system: from signaling to disease. *Antioxid Redox Signal.* 11(10):2481-504.

Spartz E. J., Freeman G. M., Jr Brown K., Farhadian B., Thienemann M., Frankovich J. 2017. Course of Neuropsychiatric Symptoms after Introduction and Removal of Nonsteroidal Anti-Inflammatory Drugs: A Pediatric Observational Study. *J. Child Adolesc. Psychopharmacol.* 27, 652-659.

Stagi S., Lepri G., Rigante D., Matucci Cerinic M., Falcini F. 2018. Cross-Sectional Evaluation of Plasma Vitamin D Levels in a Large Cohort of Italian Patients with Pediatric Autoimmune Neuropsychiatric Disorders Associated with Streptococcal Infections. *J Child Adolesc Psychopharmacol.* 28(2):124-129. doi: https://10. 1089/cap.2016.0159. Epub 2017 Nov 7. PMID: 29112476.

Stagi S., Rigante A., Lepri G., Bertini F., Matucci-Cerinic M., Falcini F. 2014. Evaluation of autoimmune phenomena in patients with pediatric autoimmune neuropsychiatric disorders associated with streptoccal infections (PANDAS). *Autoimmun Rev* 13:1236-1240.

Storch E. A., Murphy T. K., Geffken G. R., Mann G., Adkins J., Merlo L. J., Duke D., Munson M., Swaine Z., Goodman W. K. 2006. Cognitive-behavioral therapy for PANDAS-related obsessive-compulsive disorder: Findings from a preliminary waitlist controlled open trial. *J Am Acad Child Adolesc Psychiatry.* 45(10):1171-8.

Swedo S. E., Leckman J. F., Rose N. R. 2012. From research subgroup to clinical syndrome: Modifying the PANDAS criteria to describe PANS (pediatric acute-onset neuropsychiatric syndrome). *Pediatr Ther* 2:1-8.

Swedo S. E., Leonard H. L., Garvey M., Mittleman B., Allen A. J., Perlmutter S., Lougee L., Dow S., Zamkoff J., Dubbert B. K. 1998.

Pediatric autoimmune neuropsychiatric disorders associated with streptococcal infections: clinical description of the first 50 cases. *Am. J. Psychiatry* 155, 264-271.

Thienemann M., Murphy T., Leckman J., Shaw R., Williams K., Kapphahn C., Frankovich J., Geller D., Bernstein G., Chang K., Elia J., Swedo S. 2017. Clinical Management of Pediatric Acute-Onset Neuropsychiatric Syndrome: Part I- Psychiatric and Behavioral Interventions. *J. Child Adolesc. Psychopharmacol.* 27, 566-573.

Wilbur C., Bitnun A., Kronenberg S., Laxer R. M., Levy D. M., Logan W. J., Shouldice M., Yeh E. A. 2019. PANDAS/PANS in childhood: Controversies and evidence. *Paediatr Child Health.* 24(2):85-91. doi: https://10.1093/pch/pxy145. Epub 2018 Dec 9. PMID: 30996598; PMCID: PMC6462125.

Zhao Y., Jaber V., Lukiw W. J. 2017. Secretory products of the human GI tract microbiome and their potential impact on Alzheimer's disease (AD): detection of lipopolysaccharide (LPS) in AD hippocampus. *Front Cell Infect Microbiol.* 7:318.

In: Obsessive-Compulsive Disorder
Editor: Jeffrey L. Nelson

ISBN: 978-1-68507-310-7
© 2021 Nova Science Publishers, Inc.

Chapter 4

THE EFFECTS OF COVID-19 PANDEMIC ON CHILDREN AND ADOLESCENTS WITH OBSESSIVE-COMPULSIVE DISORDER

Canan Kuygun Karci[*], MD*

Department of Child and Adolescent Psychiatry,
Dr. Ekrem Tok Psychiatry Hospital, Adana, Turkey

ABSTRACT

The past one year has been difficult for people around the world in a way that has not been experienced before. Studies examining the effects of the COVID-19 pandemic are increasing day by day. It is known that traumas and difficult life events may trigger or worsen obsessive-compulsive disorder (OCD) symptoms. Numerous studies with adult OCD patients have reported that these patients are more vulnerable to COVID-19-related stress and their OCD symptoms worsened also new obsessions and compulsions developed during the COVID-19 pandemic. There are very few studies in the literature

---

[*] Corresponding Author's E-mail: c_kuy@hotmail.com.

investigating the effects of the COVID-19 pandemic on children and adolescents with OCD. In this chapter, the effects of the COVID-19 pandemic on children and adolescents with OCD will be discussed.

INTRODUCTION

The SARS-CoV-2 disease (COVID-19), which started in Wuhan, China and spread all over the world, was declared as a pandemic by the World Health Organization (WHO) on 11 March 2020. Along with the pandemic, many restrictive measures implemented to reduce the spread of the virus entered our daily lives. In line with WHO recommendations, information on how to prevent the transmission of the virus was constantly given to the general public (WHO 2020).

Attention to social distance and warnings to increase personal hygiene (especially hand hygiene) were the most important issues in reducing transmission. The protection of social distance during the pandemic process was not left to individual preference from time to time. Closing schools, restaurants, cafes and recreation centers, canceling sports and art events, curfews and even lockdowns have made social distancing mandatory. In addition to all these, millions of cases and deaths, severe economic difficulties and an increase in unemployment are among the global effects of the pandemic (WHO 2021).

Numerous studies have shown increased psychological distress, anxiety, depression, and health anxiety during the COVID-19 pandemic (Nikcevic et al., 2020, Taylor et al., 2020, Luo et al., 2020, Serafini et al., 2020). It can also be predicted that the COVID-19 pandemic will have negative effects on the mental health of children and adolescents. Even the children who did not have psychiatric complaints before the pandemic experienced psychological distress during the COVID-19 pandemic (Duan et al., 2020, Wang et al., 2020). As expected, children and adolescents with pre-existing psychiatric disease experienced more impairment than those without (Cost et al., 2021). In this chapter, the effects of the COVID-19 pandemic on children and adolescents with obsessive-compulsive disorder (OCD) will be discussed.

EFFECTS OF COVID-19 PANDEMIC ON CHILDREN AND ADOLESCENTS

Daily routines and structured daytime have great importance in maintaining the mental well-being of children and adolescents (Bridley and Jordan 2012, Brazendale et al., 2017). School and extracurricular activities contribute to manage physical activity, sleep cycle, socialization and to establish daily routine. The school closures, the suspension of social activities and curfews caused children and adolescents to spend less time outside during the COVID-19 pandemic. The stress due to the social isolation created by all these affects the mental health of children and adolescents negatively (Yeasmin et al., 2020, Cost et al., 2021).

Children and adolescents, who must stay at home, have started to spend much more time with social media/internet and technological devices (such as television, tablet, computer, mobile phone) (Duan et al., 2020). The use of the internet has inevitably increased due to getting news about the agenda, communicating with friends and/or loved ones and online education. However, many studies have shown that the children and adolescents spent significantly more time in internet by playing games and/or watching videos during the COVID-19 pandemic (Dong et al., 2020, DAK-Studie 2020, Orgiles et al., 2020). Pandemic conditions have created a serious risk in terms of problematic internet use and/or internet addiction. Additionally, it has increased the risk of children and adolescents being exposed to cyberbullying.

The anxiety and depression symptoms of children quarantined due to illness, both about their own illness and the health of their loved ones, increased during the COVID-19 pandemic (Orgiles et al., 2020). In a meta-analysis, anxiety, stress, sadness, boredom, depressive symptoms, sleep disturbance and fear were the most common emotional and behavioral problems observed in children and adolescents during the COVID-19 pandemic (Panda et al., 2021).

EFFECTS OF COVID-19 PANDEMIC ON CHILDREN AND ADOLESCENTS WITH OCD

It has been shown that OCD symptoms worsened, and health anxiety increased in previous pandemics (H1N1, Zika virus, Ebola) (Brand et al., 2013, Blakey et al., 2015, Blakey and Abramowitz 2017). Numerous studies with adult OCD patients have reported that these patients are more vulnerable to COVID-19-related stress (Samimi Ardestani et al., 2021, Khosravani et al., 2021) and their OCD symptoms worsened (Davide et al., 2020, French and Lyne 2020, Jelinek et al., 2021, Hassoulas et al., 2021), also new obsessions and compulsions developed (Benatti et al., 2020) during the COVID-19 pandemic.

Studies investigating the effects of the COVID-19 pandemic on children and adolescents with OCD are very few in the literature. In the study conducted by Tanir et al., (2020) with 61 children and adolescents diagnosed with OCD, an increase in symptom severity was found in 54.09% of the cases according to the Children's Yale-Brown Obsessive-Compulsive Scale (CY-BOCS) and Clinical Global Impression-Symptom severity (CGI-S) scores during the COVID-19 pandemic. 11.4% of the patients in the study were not receiving current treatment. 55.7% of the patients relapsed during the pandemic. While the most common symptoms were contamination obsessions and cleaning/washing compulsions before and after the pandemic, there was a significant increase in these two symptoms during the pandemic (respectively, $p = 0.008$, $p = 0.039$). A significant relationship has found between the CY-BOCS scores with talking and/or searching about COVID-19 in the social environment, daily preoccupation with COVID-19, having COVID-19 in acquaintance and the duration of OCD (Tanir et al., 2020).

Similarly, the overemphasis on handwashing, exposure to social media and environments during the pandemic has worsened the symptoms of adult patients with OCD, especially those with obsessions about contamination, cleanliness, or hygiene (Banerjee 2020, French and Lyne 2020). The study of Tanir et al., was conducted 6 weeks after the detection of first COVID-19 case in Turkey (April 2020), and all data were obtained by telephone or via online interviews.

In another early study (April-May 2020), children and adolescents were divided into two groups; survey group (n = 37) includes patients diagnosed years ago and completed primary treatment; clinical group (n = 65) includes newly diagnosed patients with current OCD treatment (Nissen, Hojgaard and Thomsen 2020). OCD, anxiety, depressive symptoms and avoidance have worsened in both groups. However, a more severe worsening in all parameters was reported in the survey group. The clinical group has easier access to psychiatric help during the pandemic, and it has been suggested that this may have a protective effect on OCD symptoms. A relationship was found between the worsening of OCD symptoms during the pandemic with the aggressive/sexual obsessions, not contamination/cleaning obsessions, poor insight at baseline, early onset of OCD and a family history of psychiatric disorders. In this study, OCD symptom severity was evaluated with a designed self-reported questionnaire.

In April-May 2020, 29 children and adolescents with OCD (diagnosed in one year) in Israel were evaluated in terms of OCD symptom severity due to COVID-19 pandemic (Schwartz-Lifshitz et al., 2021). CGI-S, CGI-I (Improvement) and Obsessive-Compulsive Inventory-Child Version (OCI-CV) were used to evaluate obsessive-compulsive symptoms. In this study, no exacerbation in OCD symptoms or increase in symptom severity during the COVID-19 pandemic was found compared to the pre-pandemic period. Even, according to the CGI-I scores, improvement in symptoms and functioning was observed in most patients during the pandemic process. All patients in the study were receiving treatment for OCD, with 42% receiving online psychotherapeutic intervention during the pandemic. It has been suggested that receiving treatment during the pandemic may have a protective effect. Both before and during the pandemic CGI-S and CGI-I scores were included in the study, but only during the pandemic OCI-CV scores were included. In addition, since the sample of this study is quite small, it reduces the effect size of the results.

Guido et al. (2021) investigated the impact of the COVID-19 pandemic on children and adolescents with pediatric autoimmune neuropsychiatric disorders associated with streptococcal infections (PANDAS) and pediatric acute-onset neuropsychiatric syndrome (PANS). A total of 108 patients aged 3-21 years with PANDAS/PANS were included in the study, which was conducted in April/May 2020. Data were obtained by a semi-structured questionnaire via online. The researchers hypothesized that lockdown would be protective against symptom worsening, as patients' exposure to viral agents would be reduced. On the contrary, increased symptoms was detected in 71% of the patients. According to the parents, the risk factors leading to this increase are the social contact reduction 78%, change or loss routine 33%, confined spaces 32%, negative family climate 30%, absence of other supports 23%, the fear of contracting the virus 18%, the suspension of psychotherapy 17% and/or drug treatment 6%. An increase in tics was observed in more than half of the patients during the lockdown. Sleep disturbances, emotional lability such as anxiety, irritability, depression, somatic complaints and new onset symptoms such as depressive mood and eating disorders, have been reported to be associated with symptom increase. A significant correlation was found between the symptom increase/new symptoms and the fear of contracting the virus. It has been suggested that parents' perception in the effectiveness of their strategies in managing children's stress during the pandemic is protective against symptom exacerbation in the child. The pre-pandemic data of the patients in the study were obtained from the parents retrospectively during the study, which may lead to recall bias.

Khan et al. (2021) investigated fear of COVID-19 and obsessive-compulsive symptoms in 63 adolescents with pre-existing psychiatric disorder. The pre-existing diagnosis was neurodevelopmental, disruptive, impulse control and conduct disorder in 42.9% of patients, mood and anxiety disorders in 36.5%, OCD in 12,7% and other diagnosis in 7.9%. 6.3% of the patients were not receiving any treatment. COVID-19 inventory and obsessive-compulsive inventory-revised (OCI-R) were used in this study. According to the COVID-19 inventory scores, 90.4% of the patients had significant worries related to the pandemic. When the patients were classified according to the COVID-19 inventory scores, significant obsessive-compulsive symptoms were reported in 85.7% of the patients in the severe category. It has been suggested that pandemic-related worries may predict the obsessive compulsive symptoms in adolescent with pre-existing psychiatric disorder.

In the literature, there is a case report of a 13-year-old adolescent with ASD who experienced OCD symptom exacerbation during the COVID-19 pandemic (Gray et al., 2021). The case developed dehydration and metabolic ketoacidosis due to increased fear of contamination and decreased oral intake, and then was feeding with a nasogastric tube. In addition to the pre-existing treatment (oxcarbazepine, clonidine and risperidone) sertraline and olanzapine were started. According to his family, these complaints started after the hospital visit of family to give COVID-19 test. This patient's OCD symptom exacerbation occurred during the COVID-19 pandemic, but it is difficult to relate it to the pandemic.

Seçer and Ulaş (2020) reported that there is a positive correlation between fear of COVID-19 and OCD symptoms, and that emotional reactivity, experiential avoidance, and depression/anxiety play a mediator role in this relationship. The sample of the study consists of 598 adolescents between 14-18 ages and all data were collected online. It was not conducted with a clinical sample, but with convenience students whose OCD symptoms were screened with the OCI-CV.

OCD symptoms were detected in 67.3% of 150 randomly selected adolescents aged 13-19 years who were questioned about their OCD symptoms with the Maudsley Obsessive Compulsive Inventory Questionnaire (Darvishi et al., 2020). The most frequent OCD symptom was washing compulsions. This study, like the study of Secer and Ulas, has a population sample and a diagnostic instrument for OCD was not used in the study.

CONCLUSION

It is obvious that the COVID-19 pandemic has negative effects on all age groups and on both healthy people and those with mental disorders. It is thought that requests for psychiatric help will increase in relation to the pandemic. Knowing thoroughly the effects of the pandemic on mental health is very important in terms of planning appropriate and effective psychiatric interventions.

Very few studies investigating the impact of the COVID-19 pandemic on children and adolescents with OCD have all been conducted in the first months of the pandemic. However, the pandemic has been going on for almost two years and it can be predicted that the acute and the chronic effect of the pandemic may be different. Therefore, longitudinal studies with large samples, using standardized measurement methods and examining the parameters such as treatment status and comorbidity are needed.

REFERENCES

Banerjee D D. 2020. The other side of COVID-19: Impact on obsessive compulsive disorder (OCD) and hoarding. *Psychiatry Res.* 288, 112966. https://doi.org/10.1016/j.psychres.2020.112966.

Benatti B, Albert U, Maina G, Fiorillo A, Celebre L, Girone N, Fineberg N, Bramante S, Rigardetto S, Dell'Osso B. 2020. What Happened to Patients With Obsessive Compulsive Disorder During the COVID-19 Pandemic? A Multicentre Report From Tertiary Clinics in Northern Italy. *Front Psychiatry.* Jul 21;11:720. doi: 10.3389/fpsyt.2020.00720. PMID: 32793008; PMCID: PMC7385249.

Blakey S M, Reuman L, Jacoby R J, Abramowitz J S. 2015. Tracing "Fearbola:" Psychological Predictors of Anxious Responding to the Threat of Ebola. *Cognit. Ther. Res.* 39(6):816-825. doi: 10.1007/s10608-015-9701-9. Epub 2015 Jun 19. PMID: 32214559; PMCID: PMC7088101.

Blakey S M, Abramowitz J S. 2017. Psychological Predictors of Health Anxiety in Response to the Zika Virus. *J. Clin. Psychol. Med. Settings.* Dec;24(3-4):270-278. doi: 10.1007/s10880-017-9514-y. PMID: 29063232; PMCID: PMC7088051.

Brand J, McKay D, Wheaton MG, Abramowitz JS. 2013. The relationship between obsessive compulsive beliefs and symptoms, anxiety and disgust sensitivity, and Swine Flu fears. *J Obsessive Compuls Relat Disord.* Apr;2(2):200-206. doi: 10.1016/j.jocrd.2013.01.007. *Epub* 2013 Mar 5. PMID: 32288994; PMCID: PMC7104149.

Brazendale K, Beets M W, Weaver R G, Pate R R, Turner-McGrievy G M, Kaczynski A T, Chandler J L, Bohnert A, von Hippel P T. 2017. Understanding differences between summer vs. school obesogenic behaviors of children: the structured days hypothesis. *Int. J. Behav. Nutr. Phys. Act.* Jul 26;14(1):100. doi: 10.1186/s12966-017-0555-2. PMID: 28747186; PMCID: PMC5530518.

Bridley A, Jordan S S. 2012. Child routines moderate daily hassles and children's psychological adjustment. *Children's Health Care* 41(2):129–144.

Cost K T, Crosbie J, Anagnostou E, Birken C S, Charach A, Monga S, Kelley E, Nicolson R, Maguire J L, Burton C L, Schachar R J, Arnold PD, Korczak DJ. 2021. Mostly worse, occasionally better: impact of COVID-19 pandemic on the mental health of Canadian children and adolescents. *Eur. Child Adolesc. Psychiatry.* Feb 26:1–14. doi: 10.1007/s00787-021-01744-3. Epub ahead of print. PMID: 33638005; PMCID: PMC7909377.

DAK-Studie. 2020. *DAK-Studie: Gaming, Social-Media & Corona.* https://www.dak.de/dak/gesundheit/dak-studie-gaming-social-media-und-corona-2295548.html.

Darvishi E, Golestan S, Demehri F, Jamalnia S. 2020. A cross-sectional study on cognitive errors and obsessive-compulsive disorders among young people during the outbreak of coronavirus disease 2019. *Activitas Nervosa Superior*, 62(4), 137-142. doi:10.1007/s41470-020-00077-x.

Davide P, Andrea P, Martina O, Andrea E, Davide D, Mario A. 2020. The impact of the COVID-19 pandemic on patients with OCD: Effects of contamination symptoms and remission state before the quarantine in a preliminary naturalistic study. *Psychiatry Res.* Sep;291:113213. doi: 10.1016/j.psychres.2020.113213. Epub 2020 Jun 9. PMID: 32535508; PMCID: PMC7280119.

Dong H, Yang F, Lu X, Hao W. 2020. Internet Addiction and Related Psychological Factors Among Children and Adolescents in China During the Coronavirus Disease 2019 (COVID-19) Epidemic. *Front Psychiatry.* Sep 2;11:00751. doi: 10.3389/fpsyt.2020.00751. PMID: 32982806; PMCID: PMC749253.

Duan L, Shao X, Wang Y, Huang Y, Miao J, Yang X, Zhu G. 2020. An investigation of mental health status of children and adolescents in china during the outbreak of COVID-19. J Affect Disord. Oct 1;275:112-118. doi: 10.1016/j.jad.2020.06.029. *Epub* 2020 Jul 2. PMID: 32658812; PMCID: PMC7329661.

French I, Lyne J. 2020. Acute exacerbation of OCD symptoms precipitated by media reports of COVID-19. Ir J Psychol Med. Dec;37(4):291-294. doi: 10.1017/ipm.2020.61. Epub 2020 May 21. PMID: 32434605; PMCID: PMC7306547.

Gray J, Bazargan-Hejazi S, Ebrahim G, Cho D. 2021. Severe OCD Exacerbation in a Patient with Autism Spectrum Disorder: A Case Report. Arch Clin Med Case Rep. 5(3):388-392. doi: 10.26502/acmcr.96550370. *Epub* 2021 May 5. PMID: 34485851; PMCID: PMC8415739.

Guido C A, Loffredo L, Zicari A M, Pavone P, Savasta S, Gagliano A, Brindisi G, Galardini G, Bertolini A, Spalice A. 2021. The Impact of the COVID-19 Epidemic During the Lockdown on Children With the Pediatric Acute-Onset Neuropsychiatric Syndrome (PANDAS/

PANS): The Importance of Environmental Factors on Clinical Conditions. *Front Neurol.* Aug 11;12:702356. doi: 10.3389/fneur. 2021.702356. PMID: 34456853; PMCID: PMC8385147.

Hassoulas A, Umla-Runge K, Zahid A, Adams O, Green M, Hassoulas A, Panayiotou E. 2021. Investigating the Association Between Obsessive-Compulsive Disorder Symptom Subtypes and Health Anxiety as Impacted by the COVID-19 Pandemic: A Cross-Sectional Study. *Psychol. Rep.* Aug 20:332941211040437. doi: 10.1177/003329 41211040437. Epub ahead of print. PMID: 34412543.

Jelinek L, Moritz S, Miegel F, Voderholzer U. 2021. Obsessive-compulsive disorder during COVID-19: Turning a problem into an opportunity? *J Anxiety Disord.* Jan;77:102329. doi: 10.1016/ j.janxdis. 2020.102329. *Epub* 2020 Nov 5. PMID: 33190017; PMCID: PMC7644184.

Khan Y S, Jouda M, Albobali Y, Osman Abouelseoud M, Souid A, AlMeraisi M J, Alabdulla M. 2021. COVID-19 pandemic fears and obsessive-compulsive symptoms in adolescents with pre-existing mental disorders: An exploratory cross-sectional study. *Clin Child Psychol Psychiatry.* May 28:13591045211017606. doi: 10.1177/ 13591045211017606. *Epub ahead of print.* PMID: 34049450.

Khosravani V, Asmundson G J G, Taylor S, Sharifi Bastan F, Samimi Ardestani S M. 2021. The Persian COVID stress scales (Persian-CSS) and COVID-19-related stress reactions in patients with obsessive-compulsive and anxiety disorders. *J. Obsessive Compuls. Relat. Disord.* Jan;28:100615. doi: 10.1016/j.jocrd.2020.100615. Epub 2020 Dec 17. PMID: 33354499; PMCID: PMC7746142.

Luo M, Guo L, Yu M, Wang H. 2020. The psychological and mental impact of coronavirus disease 2019 (COVID-19) on medical staff and general public– A systematic review and meta-analysis. *Psychiatry Res.* 291:113190. doi: 10.1016/j.psychres.2020.113190.

Nikcevic A V, Marino C, Kolubinski D C, Leach D, Spada M M. 2020. Modelling the contribution of the Big Five personality traits, health anxiety, and COVID-19 psychological distress to generalized anxiety and depressive symptoms during the COVID-19 pandemic. *Journal of Affective Disorders,* 279, 578–584. https://doi.org/10.1016/j.jad. 2020.10.053.

Nissen J B, Højgaard D R M A, Thomsen P H. 2020. The immediate effect of COVID-19 pandemic on children and adolescents with obsessive compulsive disorder. *BMC Psychiatry.* Oct 20;20(1):511. doi: 10.1186/s12888-020-02905-5. PMID: 33081741; PMCID: PMC757 3524.

Orgilés M, Morales A, Delvecchio E, Mazzeschi C, Espada J P. 2020. Immediate Psychological Effects of the COVID-19 Quarantine in Youth From Italy and Spain. *Front Psychol.* Nov 6;11:579038. doi: 10.3389/fpsyg.2020.579038. PMID: 33240167; PMCID: PMC76773 01.

Panda P K, Gupta J, Chowdhury S R, Kumar R, Meena A K, Madaan P, Sharawat I K, Gulati S. 2021. Psychological and Behavioral Impact of Lockdown and Quarantine Measures for COVID-19 Pandemic on Children, Adolescents and Caregivers: A Systematic Review and Meta-Analysis. *J. Trop. Pediatr.* Jan 29;67(1):fmaa122. doi: 10.1093/tropej/fmaa122. PMID: 33367907; PMCID: PMC7798512.

Samimi Ardestani S M, Khosravani V, Sharifi Bastan F, Baloğlu M. 2021. The Persian Version of the COVID-19 Phobia Scale (Persian-C19P-S) and the Differences in COVID-19-Related Phobic Reactions in Patients with Anxiety Disorders. *Int. J. Ment. Health Addict.* Apr 7:1-17. doi: 10.1007/s11469-021-00523-0. Epub ahead of print. PMID: 33841053; PMCID: PMC8025735.

Schwartz-Lifshitz M, Basel D, Lang C, Hertz-Palmor N, Dekel I, Zohar J, Gothelf D. 2021. Obsessive compulsive symptoms severity among children and adolescents during COVID-19 first wave in Israel. *J Obsessive Compuls Relat Disord.* Jan;28:100610. doi: 10.1016/j. jocrd.2020.100610. *Epub* 2020 Dec 2. PMID: 33288995; PMCID: PMC7709811.

Seçer İ, Ulaş S. 2020. An Investigation of the Effect of COVID-19 on OCD in Youth in the Context of Emotional Reactivity, Experiential Avoidance, Depression and Anxiety. *Int. J. Ment. Health Addict.* Jun

13:1-14. doi: 10.1007/s11469-020-00322-z. Epub ahead of print. PMID: 32837429; PMCID: PMC7293436.

Serafini G, Parmigiani B, Amerio A, Aguglia A, Sher L, Amore M. 2020. The psychological impact of COVID-19 on the mental health in the general population. *QJM.* 113:531–7. doi:10.1093/qjmed/hcaa201.

Tanir Y, Karayagmurlu A, Kaya İ, Kaynar T B, Türkmen G, Dambasan BN, Meral Y, Coşkun M. 2020. Exacerbation of obsessive-compulsive disorder symptoms in children and adolescents during COVID-19 pandemic. Psychiatry Res. Nov; 293:113363. doi: 10.1016/j.psychres. 2020.113363. *Epub 2020 Aug 3.* PMID: 32798931; PMCID: PMC7837048.

Taylor S, Landry C A, Paluszek M M, Rachor G S, Asmundson G J. 2020. Worry, avoidance, and coping during the COVID-19 pandemic: A comprehensive network analysis. *Journal of Anxiety Disorders*, 76, 102327. https://doi.org/10.1016/j.janxdis. 2020.102327.

Wang Y, Zhao X, Feng Q, Liu L, Yao Y, Shi J. 2020. Psychological assistance during the coronavirus disease 2019 outbreak in China. *J. Health Psychol.* 733–737.

World Health Organization. 2020. *Novel coronavirus (2019-nCoV):* Situation report, 19.

World Health Organization. 2021. *Coronavirus Disease (COVID-19) Dashboard.* WHO, January 12. covid19.who.int.

Yeasmin S, Banik R, Hossain S, Hossain M N, Mahumud R, Salma N, Hossain MM. 2020. Impact of COVID-19 pandemic on the mental health of children in Bangladesh: A cross-sectional study. *Child Youth Serv. Rev.* Oct;117:105277. doi: 10.1016/j.childyouth. 2020.105277. *Epub 2020 Jul 29.* PMID: 32834275; PMCID: PMC7387938.

In: Obsessive-Compulsive Disorder
Editor: Jeffrey L. Nelson

ISBN: 978-1-68507-310-7
© 2021 Nova Science Publishers, Inc.

Chapter 5

A REVIEW OF CONSIDERATIONS IN ASSESSING AND TREATING RELIGIOUS-THEMED OBSESSIONS

Kelly N. Banneyer[*], *PhD*

Department of Pediatrics, Baylor College of Medicine,
Houston, Texas, USA

ABSTRACT

OCD oftentimes can target an individual's values. For those individuals of a strong faith background, scrupulosity can become a focus of intrusive thoughts. Scrupulosity may involve intrusive thoughts related to blasphemy, having committed a sin, behaving morally, purity, going to Hell, death, or a loss of control. 24.8% of adults and 37.7% of children with OCD have religious obsessions, and these obsessions can vary across religious groups. Compulsions associated with these behaviors can include confessing, seeking reassurance, cleansing and purifying rituals, excessive prayer, and avoidance of triggers. This

---

[*] Corresponding Author's E-mail: knbanney@texaschildrens.org.

chapter will explain the role that religion takes in certain presentations of OCD and inform clinicians how to differentiate between standard religious practices and compulsive behaviors. In working within an exposure-based cognitive behavioral model for intervention, this chapter will also discuss implications for evidence-based treatment using a case example.

Keywords: obsessive-compulsive disorder; scrupulosity; exposure and response prevention

INTRODUCTION

Obsessive-compulsive disorder (OCD) involves the presence of obsessions and/or compulsions that are present and interfere in functioning for at least one hour per day in children and two hours per day in adults (American Psychiatric Association [APA] 2013). Obsessions can take a variety of themes. According to the Yale-Brown Obsessive Compulsive Scale (Goodman et al., 1989), a checklist and severity scale commonly used to diagnose OCD, common themes of obsessions include the following: aggressive, contamination, sexual, hoarding/saving, religious (scrupulosity), and need for symmetry or exactness. This chapter will focus on religious obsessions as this occurrence is more common than treatment providers often believe, and important multicultural considerations are indicated when working with religious-themed obsessions.

This chapter is intended for the scientific community, in addition to treatment providers and learners, to obtain a better understanding of the implications of scrupulosity-based obsessions and implications on intervention and assessment based on research findings and clinical practice. This chapter will first discuss the presentation of scrupulosity-themed obsessions along with common compulsions, will give a review of related research, will discuss assessment and intervention implications from a multicultural framework, and will finally provide a case example.

UNDERSTANDING OCD AND SCRUPULOSITY

Suspected instances of scrupulosity were documented as early as the 16th century. For example, the religious figure Martin Luther was believed to fear that he would omit statements during mass indicative of sinful behavior. In response to this obsessive fear, he demonstrated compulsive confessing multiple times each day. Additionally, in the 17th century, John Bunyan experienced obsessive fear of blasphemy triggered by thoughts that were homicidal or sexual in nature. Because of this, he engaged in compulsions of "undoing." Other religious figures believed to experience scrupulosity-themed OCD were St. Ignatius Loyola, St. Veronica Giullani, and St. Alphonsus Liguori (Cefalu 2010; Pollard 2010).

OCD is oftentimes described as a computer virus in that it attacks the vulnerable parts of the mind, or the beliefs and values of an individual. Obsessions related to scrupulosity may take themes of blasphemy, having committed a sin, behaving morally, purity, going to Hell, death, or a loss of impulse control. Related behavioral compulsions may include the following: excessive trips to confession, repeatedly seeking reassurance from religious leaders and loved ones, repeated cleansing and purifying rituals, acts of self-sacrifice, and avoiding situations (for example, religious services) in which one believes a religious or moral error would be especially likely or cause something bad to happen. Related mental compulsions may include the following: excessive praying (sometimes with an emphasis on the prayer needing to be perfect), repeatedly imagining sacred images or phrases, repeating passages from sacred scriptures in one's head, and making pacts with God.

Clarifying the designation between normative religious practice and compulsive behaviors can be difficult. Many religions have ritualized behaviors that are expected to be performed (such as praying in a certain way at specific times of the day). However, these behaviors are not indicative of OCD unless they exceed cultural norms, are deemed inappropriate by others of the same culture, or interfere with the individuals' functioning (Cefalu 2010). An expert in the field described that "unlike normal religious practice, scrupulous behavior usually exceeds or disregards religious law and may focus excessively on one trivial area of religious practice while other, more important areas may be completely ignored. The behavior of scrupulous individuals is typically inconsistent with that of the rest of the faith community" (Pollard 2010 p.1). Several points have been highlighted to help determine the difference between normative religious practice and behaviors associated with OCD. If behavior goes beyond the requirements of religious law, has a narrow focus, focuses on trivial components of religious practice, or involves scruples that interpret religious text as absolute mandates, it may be indicative of OCD (Ciarrocchi 1995). Having a concerete understanding of these differences is important for valid and reliable diagnosis and subsequent treatment planning.

A Review of Research:
Prevalence and Presentation

The overall 12-month incidence rate of OCD in the United States among adults is 1.2% (Kessler 2005). This rate is higher for females (1.8%) than for males (0.5%), and rates tend to decrease as age progresses (estimated at 1.5% for 18-29 year olds, 1.4% for 30-44 year olds, 1.1% for 45-59 year olds, and 0.5% for individuals over age 60; 2005). Prevalence rates for children are usually estimated as 0.5-2.0% (Eichstedt & Arnold 2001). Looking specifically at scrupulosity, 24.8% of adults and 37.7% of children with OCD were found to have religious obsessions in the United States, and there were no differences between genders (Hunt 2020). Looking globally, researchers found that 24.8% of adults with OCD experience religious obsessions in the USA and Europe, 28.6% in South Africa, 32.7% in the Middle East, 19.4% in Asia, and 31.9% in South America (Hunt 2020).

Generally, a recent meta-analysis found that rates of specific presentations of OCD are more similar across ages, genders, and cultures than previously thought and reported (Hunt 2020). When looking at predictive factors, it has been established that spirituality and religion do not cause or predict OCD (Abramowitz & Buchholz, 2020). In fact, almost one out of every five adults who experience obsessions of scrupulosity report they do not have a religious affiliation (Siev et al., 2011). However some researchers have demonstrated the degree of scrupulosity in patients with OCD does differ across religious affiliation. For instance, in a sample of Catholic, Protestant, Jewish, and non-religious individuals, Catholic individuals had higher levels of scrupulosity than Jewish and non-religious individuals (Buchholz et al., 2019). In looking at adults with OCD, those who experience religious-themed obsessions were overall more religious, more likely to seek counseling from a religious figure, less likely to seek medication for relief of OCD symptoms, and more likely to report that OCD symptoms interfered with faith and religious practice in comparison to those adults with OCD who did not experience religious obsessions (Siev et al. 2011).

Research does seem consistent in reporting that specific obsessions may differ in themes between different religious faiths. For example, on a scale measuring fears of sin and punishment from God, devout Jews were found to demonstrate fewer fears in comparison to devout Catholics and Protestants (Abramowitz et al. 2002). Additionally, Huppert and colleagues (2007) reported Christians are more likely to have obsessions regarding worshipping the Devil or going to Hell while Orthodox Jews may be more likely to experience obsessions related to following religious practices correctly regarding cleanliness, purity, or prayer.

Additionally, researchers have found that the presence of scrupulosity-themed intrusive thoughts predicts poorer outcomes in OCD treatment (Abramowitz & Buchholz 2020). This may be related to provider knowledge (or lack thereof) of scrupulosity-related OCD and differentiating symptoms from normative religious practices. Overall it seems that being devout or following a specific religion does not predict incidence of OCD, but for individuals with OCD, those who are religious may experience scrupulosity-themed obsessions and/or compulsions, and this may have treatment implications.

ASSESSMENT AND INTERVENTION IMPLICATIONS

Assessment

As mentioned above, for the assessment and diagnosis of OCD, the gold standard assessment measure in adults is the Yale–Brown Obsessive Compulsive Scale (Y-BOCS; Goodman et al., 1989). One specific measure does exist to measure scrupulosity symptoms, the Penn Inventory of Scrupulosity (PIOS; Olatunji et al., 2007). The PIOS is a 19-item self-report scale for adults. The measure consists of two subscales (validated with factor analysis) that measure fears about having committed a sin and about punishment from God. It was found to have good convergent and discriminate validity (Abramowitz et al., 2002). This measure can be used for clinical or research purposes.

Intervention

The gold standard evidence-based intervention for treating OCD is exposure and response prevention (see Storch et al. 2019), and this continues to be the case with patients presenting with religious-themed obsessions and associated compulsions (see Siev et al. 2020). Exposure and response prevention follows the model that compulsive behaviors result as a means to nullify uncomfortable feelings. This posits from cognitive behavioral theory. For instance, when an individual experiences an obsession, this is associated with uncomfortable feelings, such as anxiety or disgust. To reduce these negative feelings, an individual with OCD engages in a compulsive behavior that temporarily results in relief from discomfort. However, these compulsive behaviors interfere in functioning and are not adaptive. Over time, compulsive behaviors can increase or become repetitive as individuals try to find continued and ongoing relief from uncomfortable feelings that accompany obsessive thoughts. Exposure and response prevention is an intervention that involves exposing an individual to a stimulus that triggers an obsessive thought without the individual engaging in the learned compulsion. This results in new learning that the individual is able to tolerate uncomfortable feelings.

Completing exposure and response prevention with individuals with scrupulosity requires a multicultural framework. As indicated above, most individuals who present with religious-themed OCD do identify with a particular religion. Navigating a balance between reducing and eliminating compulsions while still allowing the individual to practice their faith with typical practices can be difficult to do. The therapist working with a person impacted by OCD must have a good understanding of religious practices, and this may involve consulting with the individual, the individual's family, or religious figures. The goal is for the individual to engage in behaviors opposed to those dictated by OCD while still being able to follow religious practices (see Huppert et al. 2007). For instance, some religions constitute that individuals do not experience doubt and instead operate completely with faith in God. However, oftentimes OCD is conceptualized as the "doubting disease," and experiencing uncertainty may be a treatment goal. The therapist may need to work with the family to determine how to potentially limit or eliminate prayer and confession if these are compulsive behaviors outside typical religious practice that are interfering in the individual's functioning.

CASE EXAMPLE

"Emma" was a 19 year old who identified as a Caucasian, cisgender female of the Catholic faith. She presented to treatment with obsessions of scrupulosity, in particular fears that she was going to Hell, had been possessed, and would procreate with the Devil. These obsessions were associated with compulsions of excessive, repetitive prayer, and avoidance of specific triggers (books and television shows that featured possession or demons). During the diagnostic intake, it was determined that Emma was the product of a typical birth and delivery. She experienced typical development and demonstrated above average cognitive abilities, as evidenced by her maintaining high grades and enrollment in a university program. As a child and teenager, Emma had experienced some anxiety symptoms, such as perfectionism and the desire to please others. Socially, Emma had an intact family, and she was involved in multiple organizations through her school and church. Emma identified that the onset of her obsessive thoughts occurred in high school when she attended a mass where the concept of possession was discussed. Emma then began to experience the concern that she had been possessed and started to engage in compulsive behavior to negate this concern. At first, Emma met with her priest and with a religious counselor, but her OCD symptoms continued to interfere with her daily functioning, with an estimated three hours per day occupied by obsessions and compulsions. According to the Y-BOCS, Emma's severity was in the moderate range, and she demonstrated obsessions in the domain of scrupulosity and compulsions in the domains of repetitive prayer, reassurance-seeking, and avoidance.

Emma was diagnosed with OCD, and her therapist worked to engage her in exposure and response prevention. A hierarchy of triggers was created. Emma was able to be exposed to low anxiety-provoking levels of the hierarchy without engaging in compulsive prayer during session. The therapist worked with Emma and her priest to create higher levels on the hierarchy and practices for exposure and response preventionwithout breaking religious law. For example, Emma indicated that she would be able to limit her prayer each day, but praying to the Devil would not be in accordance with her religious values. Emma was able to engage in exposure practice in therapy sessions and in her home and school environments. Emma also requested a family-based session so that her family members could understand the function of OCD and how they could help in treatment by limiting accommodation and reassurance. After twelve weeks of intervention services, Emma showed significant improvement in functioning and much decreased symptoms of OCD.

CONCLUSION

Religious-themed obsessions, or obsessions of scrupulosity, are common in individuals suffering from OCD. However, this domain is often met with confusion or ignorance form researchers and treatment providers. This chapter sought to give an overview of common presentations of scrupulosity-based OCD, describe research findings regarding prevalence and presentation, discuss assessment and treatment implications, and provide a case example. Researchers and treatment providers who work with individuals with OCD should be aware of the differences between normative religious practice and potentially compulsive and interfering behaviors. Additionally, consultation with religious figures may be necessary to better understand these differences and work with this population.

REFERENCES

Abramowitz, J. S., & Buchholz, J. L. (2020). Spirituality/religion and obsessive–compulsive-related disorders. *Handbook of Spirituality, Religion, and Mental Health*, 61-78.

American Psychiatric Association. 2013. *Diagnostic and statistical manual of mental disorders: DSM-5*. Arlington, VA: American Psychiatric Association.

Buchholz, J. L., Abramowitz, J. S., Riemann, B. C., Reuman, L., Blakey, S. M., Leonard, R. C., & Thompson, K. A. (2019). Scrupulosity, religious affiliation and symptom presentation in obsessive compulsive disorder. *Behavioural and cognitive psychotherapy*, *47*(4), 478-492.

Cefalu, P. (2010). The doubting disease: Religious scrupulosity and obsessive-compulsive disorder in historical context. *Journal of Medical Humanities*, *31*(2), 111-125.

Ciarrocchi, J. W. (1995). *The doubting disease: Help for scrupulosity and religious compulsions*. Paulist Press.

Eichstedt, Julie A., and Sharon L. Arnold. "Childhood-onset obsessive-compulsive disorder: a tic-related subtype of OCD?." *Clinical psychology review* 21, no. 1 (2001): 137-157.

Goodman, Wayne K., Lawrence H. Price, Steven A. Rasmussen, Carolyn Mazure, Roberta L. Fleischmann, Candy L. Hill, George R. Heninger, and Dennis S. Charney. "The Yale-Brown obsessive compulsive scale: I. Development, use, and reliability." *Archives of general psychiatry* 46, no. 11 (1989): 1006-1011.

Hunt, Christopher. "Differences in OCD symptom presentations across age, culture, and gender: A quantitative review of studies using the Y-BOCS symptom checklist." *Journal of Obsessive-Compulsive and Related Disorders* 26 (2020): 100533.

Huppert, J. D., Siev, J., & Kushner, E. S. (2007). When religion and obsessive–compulsive disorder collide: Treating scrupulosity in ultra-orthodox Jews. *Journal of Clinical Psychology*, *63*(10), 925-941.

Kessler, Ronald C., Wai Tat Chiu, Olga Demler, and Ellen E. Walters. "Prevalence, severity, and comorbidity of 12-month DSM-IV disorders in the National Comorbidity Survey Replication." *Archives of general psychiatry* 62, no. 6 (2005): 617-627.

Olatunji, Bunmi O., Jonathan S. Abramowitz, Nathan L. Williams, Kevin M. Connolly, and Jeffrey M. Lohr. "Scrupulosity and obsessive-compulsive symptoms: Confirmatory factor analysis and validity of the Penn Inventory of Scrupulosity." *Journal of Anxiety Disorders* 21, no. 6 (2007): 771-787.

Pollard, C. A. (2010). Scrupulosity. Retrieved from https://iocdf.org/wp-content/uploads/2014/10/IOCDF-Scrupulosity-Fact-Sheet.pdf.

Siev, J., Baer, L., & Minichiello, W. E. (2011). Obsessive-compulsive disorder with predominantly scrupulous symptoms: Clinical and religious characteristics. *Journal of Clinical Psychology*, *67*(12), 1188-1196.

Siev, Jedidiah, Jonathan D. Huppert, and Shelby E. Zuckerman. "Understanding and treating scrupulosity." *The Wiley handbook of obsessive compulsive disorders* (2017): 527-546.

Storch, Eric A., Dean McKay, and Jonathan S. Abramowitz, eds. *Advanced casebook of obsessive-compulsive and related disorders: conceptualizations and treatment.* Academic Press, 2019.

INDEX

A

acts of aggression, 4, 8
acute-onset, v, vii, ix, 89, 90, 91, 92, 94, 101, 103, 104, 106, 107, 108, 109, 116
ADHD, 6, 13, 14, 21, 95
adolescents, vi, vii, x, 50, 86, 111, 112, 113, 114, 115, 116, 117, 118, 119, 120, 121, 122, 123
adulthood, viii, 2, 4, 6, 15, 90
adults, x, 29, 46, 125, 126, 128, 129, 130
adverse effects, 26, 99
adverse event, 25, 30
affective disorder, 14, 41
anterior cingulate cortex, 3, 19, 30, 39
antibiotic, 97, 99, 100, 107
antidepressants, viii, 2, 24, 41, 45
anti-inflammatory drugs, 101
antimicrobial therapy, 96
antipsychotic, 27, 36, 38
antipsychotic drugs, 27, 38
anxiety, vii, viii, x, 1, 2, 4, 5, 7, 9, 10, 12, 13, 24, 25, 34, 35, 36, 37, 38, 39, 40, 41, 42, 45, 53, 80, 81, 84, 86, 90, 92, 95, 112, 113, 114, 115, 116, 117, 119, 121, 122, 123, 130, 132, 134
anxiety disorder, viii, 2, 9, 12, 13, 34, 36, 38, 39, 40, 41, 45, 81, 117, 121
autoantibodies, 39, 93, 108
autoimmune, v, viii, ix, 2, 3, 6, 15, 16, 36, 89, 90, 92, 93, 95, 102, 103, 104, 105, 106, 107, 108, 109, 110, 116
autoimmune disease, 16, 36
autoimmunity, 14
avoidance, x, 24, 25, 60, 77, 80, 115, 117, 123, 125, 131

B

bacterial infection, 90
basal ganglia, 15, 16, 17, 18, 19, 37, 46, 93, 102, 105
behavior therapy, 80, 84, 96
behavioral models, 59
behavioral problems, 114
behavioral theory, 60, 130
behaviors, x, 5, 8, 10, 11, 18, 92, 119, 125, 127, 130, 131, 133
bipolar disorder, 3, 4, 6, 35

Index

blasphemy, x, 125, 127
brain, viii, 2, 18, 19, 21, 23, 37, 39, 41, 42, 46, 107, 108

C

central nervous system, 109
cerebral cortex, 17, 18
cerebrospinal fluid, 3, 21
childhood, 4, 6, 14, 68, 80, 90, 105, 108, 110
children, vi, vii, viii, ix, x, 2, 11, 14, 15, 29, 45, 46, 86, 90, 93, 94, 95, 97, 105, 106, 108, 111, 112, 113, 114, 115, 116, 118, 119, 120, 122, 123, 125, 126, 128
chorea, x, 15, 19, 90, 92, 93, 95, 101, 102, 108
citalopram, 25, 27, 42, 43
cleaning, 8, 62, 68, 114, 115
clients, 70, 71, 74, 78
clinical assessment, 33
clinical judgment, 71
clinical presentation, 58
clinical psychology, 40
clinical syndrome, 109
cognitive abilities, 132
cognitive models, 59
cognitive process, 19, 59, 72, 75
cognitive processing, 19, 75
cognitive style, 63, 69
cognitive theory, 75, 85
cognitive therapy, 71, 85
cognitive-behavioral therapy (CBT), 3, 22, 28, 29, 61, 63, 78, 96, 99, 100, 107
community, 33, 80, 85, 101, 103, 126, 128
comorbidity, viii, 2, 4, 5, 6, 7, 8, 11, 14, 15, 32, 33, 34, 35, 36, 118, 134
compulsions, v, viii, ix, x, 1, 4, 7, 8, 10, 11, 13, 15, 16, 25, 57, 58, 62, 63, 65, 71, 75, 81, 111, 114, 117, 125, 126, 127, 129, 130, 131, 134

compulsive behaviors, vii, viii, xi, 2, 4, 7, 126, 127, 130, 131
compulsive personality disorder, 9, 13
contamination, 4, 7, 8, 68, 114, 115, 117, 120, 126
controlled studies, 5, 29, 100
controlled trials, 24, 41, 46, 98, 99
cortico-striatal-thalamic-cortical dysfunction, 19
COVID-19, vi, vii, x, 16, 37, 47, 48, 49, 51, 55, 111, 112, 113, 114, 115, 116, 117, 118, 119, 120, 121, 122, 123
cross-sectional study, 120, 121, 123

D

deep brain stimulation, 3, 19, 23
depression, viii, x, 2, 3, 4, 14, 28, 31, 38, 42, 54, 80, 90, 92, 112, 113, 116, 117, 122
depressive symptoms, 25, 113, 115, 122
detection, 30, 110, 115
diagnostic criteria, vii, x, 10, 34, 90, 91, 94, 100
disability, vii, viii, 2, 4, 29
disgust, 68, 76, 82, 119, 130
disorder, vii, viii, 1, 2, 3, 4, 5, 6, 7, 8, 9, 12, 14, 15, 19, 23, 32, 33, 34, 35, 36, 37, 38, 39, 40, 41, 42, 43, 45, 46, 50, 51, 53, 54, 55, 58, 62, 72, 84, 85, 92, 95, 102, 105, 106, 107, 108, 117, 118, 121, 122, 126, 133, 134
dissociative disorders, 34
distress, 5, 8, 10, 12, 59, 61, 112
dopamine, viii, 2, 5, 17, 20, 39, 93, 102
dopaminergic, 17, 18, 20, 21
dosage, 22, 24, 25, 26, 27, 28
dose-response relationship, 42
double-blind trial, 43
drug interaction, 22
drug treatment, 11, 12, 116

drugs, 24, 27, 44

E

eating disorders, 116
egodystonia, 7
emergency, 47, 48, 49, 51, 55
emotional processes, 77, 78
endothelial dysfunction, 101
environmental factors, 65
environments, 115, 132
exacerbation, 91, 94, 95, 97, 99, 115, 116, 117, 120, 123
executive function, 17, 64
executive functioning, 64
exposure, xi, 3, 22, 29, 59, 61, 68, 73, 74, 76, 82, 84, 85, 86, 87, 115, 116, 126, 130, 131, 132
exposure and response prevention (ERP), 3, 22, 29, 46, 59, 61, 62, 63, 69, 71, 73, 76, 78, 79, 85, 86, 126, 130, 131, 132

F

factor analysis, 130, 134
faith, x, 70, 74, 76, 125, 128, 129, 131
family history, 24, 115
family members, 12, 132
fear, 13, 25, 29, 68, 73, 114, 116, 117, 127
fluoxetine, 25, 27, 28, 42
fluvoxamine, 23, 28, 41, 42
food intake, 91, 92
frontal cortex, 18, 38
frontal lobe, 21
functional MRI, 37
fusion, 60, 66, 74, 82, 83, 86

G

generalized anxiety disorder, 12

H

glutamate, viii, 2, 20, 21, 28, 40

habituation, 60, 73
health, 12, 45, 112, 113, 114, 121
heterogeneity, viii, 2, 12, 22, 62, 85
history, 11, 14, 54, 69, 75
hypothesis, 18, 107, 119

I

immune function, 36
immune response, 90, 94
immune system, 90
immunobiology, 106
immunoglobulin, 98, 105
immunomodulatory, 98
individuals, vii, ix, x, 5, 10, 11, 13, 14, 16, 23, 25, 50, 51, 54, 55, 58, 59, 61, 62, 63, 64, 68, 69, 74, 75, 77, 78, 82, 125, 127, 128, 129, 130, 131, 133
infection, ix, 3, 6, 33, 90, 91, 92, 94, 96, 97, 99, 101, 104, 105, 106, 107, 108
inflammation, 93, 105
inflammatory disease, 93
integration, 19, 29, 30, 63, 78
intervention, xi, 29, 30, 115, 126, 130, 132
intrusive thoughts, vii, viii, x, 1, 4, 7, 75, 125, 129
issues, 7, 34, 36, 62, 82, 112

L

learners, 126
learning, 17, 70, 71, 131
left hemisphere, 19
lifetime, vii, 1, 4, 5, 14, 15
limbic loop, 18
limbic system, 16, 19

longitudinal study, 95

M

major depression, viii, 2, 4, 42
management, viii, 2, 5, 9, 23, 27, 31, 55, 96
media, 113, 115, 119, 120
medical, 9, 11, 45, 54, 92, 121
medication, 5, 9, 11, 22, 23, 28, 33, 81, 96, 129
mental actions, 59
mental disorder, 80, 107, 118, 121, 133
mental health, 15, 49, 52, 54, 69, 79, 83, 112, 113, 118, 119, 120, 123, 133
mental illness, 16, 54, 55
meta-analysis, 30, 39, 40, 41, 45, 46, 62, 113, 121, 128
motor loop, 16, 17, 18
movement disorders, 31, 93, 100, 102, 104
multidimensional, 33, 83

N

nasogastric tube, 117
negative consequences, 19
negative effects, 112, 118
negative experiences, 70
negative reinforcement, 59, 69, 78
neurobiology, viii, 2, 12, 39
neurodegenerative diseases, 101
neuroimaging, 10, 19
neuroinflammation, 93, 98
neurologic symptom, 97
neuronal circuits, 18
neurons, 17, 18, 19
neuropeptides, 20
neurophysiology, 38
neuropsychiatry, 53
neuropsychopharmacology, 40
neuroscience, 44
neurosurgery, 46

neurotransmission, viii, 2, 17, 20
neurotransmitters, 20, 39
non-steroidal anti-inflammatory drugs, 98

O

obsessions, v, vi, viii, ix, x, 1, 4, 7, 8, 10, 11, 12, 13, 15, 24, 28, 29, 31, 57, 58, 62, 63, 65, 68, 69, 71, 72, 74, 75, 77, 81, 85, 111, 114, 115, 125, 126, 127, 128, 129, 130, 131, 133
obsessive-compulsive disorder (OCD), 1, iii, v, vi, vii, viii, ix, x, 1, 2, 3, 4, 5, 6, 7, 8, 9, 10, 11, 12, 13, 14, 15, 16, 18, 19, 20, 21, 22, 23, 24, 25, 26, 27, 28, 29, 30, 31, 32, 33, 34, 35, 36, 37, 38, 39, 40, 41, 42, 43, 44, 45, 46, 53, 55, 57, 58, 60, 61, 62, 63, 64, 65, 66, 68, 69, 71, 73, 74, 75, 76, 78, 79, 80, 81, 82, 83, 84, 85, 86, 87, 89, 90, 91, 92, 93, 94, 95, 97, 99, 100, 101, 104, 106, 107, 109, 111, 113, 114, 115, 117, 118, 120, 121, 122, 123, 125, 126, 127, 128, 129, 130, 131, 132, 133, 134, 135
OCD refractory, 6

P

pathophysiology, viii, ix, 2, 16, 18, 28, 31, 35, 38, 39, 90, 91, 93, 94, 98
pediatric acute-onset neuropsychiatric syndrome (PANS), v, vii, ix, 89, 90, 91, 92, 93, 94, 95, 96, 97, 98, 99, 100, 101, 102, 103, 104, 105, 107, 108, 109, 110, 116, 120
pediatric autoimmune neuropsychiatric disorders associated with streptococcal infections (PANDAS), vii, viii, ix, 2, 3, 6, 15, 90, 91, 92, 93, 94, 95, 96, 97, 98, 99, 100, 101, 102, 103, 105, 107, 108, 109, 110, 116, 120

penicillin, 96, 103, 108
perfectionism, 13, 67, 132
personal values, 75
personality, 121
personality traits, 121
pharmacotherapy, 22, 23, 41, 44
placebo, 23, 29, 41, 42, 43, 44, 45, 97, 106
population, ix, 2, 14, 19, 29, 36, 118, 123, 133
prayer, x, 125, 127, 129, 131, 132
prevention, 3, 22, 25, 29, 42, 59, 61, 73, 81, 82, 84, 85, 86, 87, 126, 130, 131, 132
prophylactic, 99, 101
prophylaxis, 97, 100, 103, 108
psychiatric disorder, viii, 2, 5, 6, 12, 19, 31, 46, 115, 116
psychiatric illness, vii, 1, 4, 31
psychiatry, ix, 2, 31, 40, 41, 42, 43, 44, 45, 46, 53, 134
psychological distress, 112, 121
psychopathology, 15, 46, 69
psychopharmacology, 40, 42, 43, 44, 86
psychosis, 50, 51, 54, 55
psychosocial functioning, 25, 42
psychosocial interventions, 5
psychosocial stress, 91
psychotherapy, 5, 29, 61, 72, 77, 80, 82, 84, 116, 133
punishment, viii, 2, 69, 129, 130
purity, x, 125, 127, 129

R

receptor, 5, 17, 20, 21, 28, 39, 40, 93
recommendations, iv, 42, 63, 96, 98, 112
relevance, 67, 68, 70, 75, 77, 78
relief, 59, 129, 130
religion, vii, xi, 126, 129, 131, 133, 134
religiosity, 58, 66, 69, 82, 83, 86
religious beliefs, 77

remission, 22, 40, 61, 62, 63, 69, 73, 74, 95, 99, 120
researchers, 58, 64, 69, 72, 75, 100, 116, 128, 129, 133
resistance, viii, 2, 14, 29, 60
response, viii, 2, 3, 5, 6, 8, 10, 11, 12, 14, 15, 19, 20, 22, 24, 25, 26, 27, 28, 29, 30, 31, 40, 41, 42, 59, 61, 62, 73, 81, 82, 83, 84, 85, 86, 87, 99, 126, 127, 130, 131, 132
risk, viii, 2, 5, 16, 24, 26, 36, 42, 73, 113, 116

S

safety, 4, 8, 25, 29, 31, 41, 42
schizophrenia, 4, 15, 36
school, x, 90, 92, 95, 112, 113, 119, 132
school performance, x, 90, 92, 95
scrupulosity, v, ix, x, 57, 58, 62, 65, 66, 68, 70, 74, 76, 79, 125, 126, 127, 128, 129, 130, 131, 133, 134, 135
selective serotonin reuptake inhibitor, 38, 43, 99
sensitivity, 68, 74, 76, 82, 104, 119
serotonin, viii, 2, 3, 5, 20, 23, 24, 25, 32, 36, 38, 39, 41, 43, 44, 80
sertraline, 23, 25, 27, 42, 117
sleep disturbance, 92, 114
social activities, 113
social anxiety, 24, 42
social distance, 112
social environment, 114
social impairment, 7
social interaction, 12
social phobia, 12, 42
stimulation, viii, 2, 3, 19, 23, 30, 41, 46
stress, x, 5, 94, 101, 105, 106, 111, 113, 114, 116, 121
stress reactions, 121
stressful life events, 54

striatum, viii, 2, 17, 18, 19, 30, 65
structure, 17, 19, 34, 35, 78
suicidal behavior, 5, 14
suicide, viii, 2, 5, 14
suicide attempts, 14
symmetry, viii, 2, 4, 7, 8, 15, 68, 126
symptom severity, 37, 97, 114, 115
symptoms, viii, ix, x, 2, 4, 6, 7, 8, 9, 11, 14, 15, 16, 18, 19, 20, 22, 23, 24, 25, 29, 30, 36, 59, 61, 62, 66, 68, 72, 74, 75, 80, 82, 83, 86, 90, 91, 92, 93, 94, 95, 97, 98, 99, 105, 108, 111, 113, 114, 115, 116, 117, 119, 120, 121, 122, 123, 129, 130, 132, 134
syndrome, vii, viii, ix, 2, 7, 9, 15, 16, 33, 36, 90, 91, 92, 101, 103, 104, 105, 107, 108, 109, 116
systemic lupus erythematosus, 16, 92

T

techniques, 29, 60, 63, 71, 77, 78, 79, 83
therapeutic effect, 41
therapeutic use, 23
therapist, 78, 131, 132
therapy, viii, 2, 22, 24, 31, 45, 63, 71, 74, 75, 80, 81, 83, 84, 85, 86, 87, 99, 109, 132
thoughts, vii, viii, x, 1, 4, 5, 7, 8, 10, 12, 13, 14, 19, 25, 29, 30, 59, 63, 66, 69, 70, 72, 75, 78, 82, 125, 127, 129, 130, 132
tic disorder, 7, 11, 14, 15, 22, 33, 91, 92, 94, 100
tics, ix, 8, 11, 15, 21, 40, 90, 92, 95, 105, 116
transcranial magnetic stimulation (TMS), viii, 2, 3, 23, 30, 41, 46
trauma, 68, 69, 74, 80
traumatic experiences, 75
treatment, vii, viii, ix, x, xi, 2, 4, 5, 6, 9, 10, 12, 13, 14, 15, 20, 22, 23, 24, 25, 26, 27, 28, 29, 30, 31, 32, 35, 36, 37, 38, 39, 40, 41, 42, 43, 44, 45, 46, 53, 55, 58, 59, 61, 62, 63, 64, 65, 66, 69, 70, 71, 74, 76, 78, 79, 80, 81, 82, 86, 90, 96, 97, 98, 100, 102, 103, 105, 107, 114, 115, 117, 118, 126, 128, 129, 131, 132, 133, 135
trial, 24, 41, 43, 44, 45, 83, 85, 86, 107, 109
trichotillomania, 9, 12
tricyclic antidepressant, 3, 25
tumor necrosis factor, 16, 95

U

underlying mechanisms, 69, 74
upper respiratory tract, 96